Intermittent Fasting

The Complete Guide for Weight Loss, Prevention and Treatment of Chronic Diseases, Healthy Lifestyle, Which Includes Diet Basics, 28 Days Meal Plan with Recipes and Shopping List

Ashley Fiorentini

Contents

Introduction

I want to thank you and congratulate you for purchasing the book, "*Intermittent Fasting*".

This book contains information on intermittent fasting. Intermittent fasting is a pattern of eating where a person cycles between periods of fasting and eating. There are several types of intermittent fasting.

Intermittent fasting has many benefits as will be discussed in this book. It helps with weight loss and lowering the levels of both insulin and blood sugar.

Some of the topics covered in this book include:

- What is Intermittent Fasting?
- Who can Fast?
- Who cannot Fast?
- Foods to Eat/Avoid
- Myths About Intermittent Fasting
- Mistakes to Avoid While on Intermittent Fasting
- Tips and Tricks for a Successful Intermittent Fasting
- 28-Day Intermittent Fasting Plan...and Many More

Thanks again for purchasing this book. Enjoy reading!

Chapter 1: Introduction to Intermittent Fasting

What is Intermittent Fasting?

Intermittent fasting is an eating pattern where a person cycles between eating and fasting periods. Therefore, it is more of a way of eating than a diet.

There are different types of intermittent fasting with each method splitting the day or week into periods of eating and fasting. Some common methods of intermittent fasting include time-restricted eating, 24-hour fasts, and alternate day fasting.

Many people report having more energy when fasting. Although hunger can be a challenge, it is manageable and will gradually become easier as your body adapts to longer periods of fasting.

Besides helping with weight loss, fasting has been shown to reduce blood sugar and insulin levels. Fasting can also increase human growth hormone, improve brain function, and may even help us live longer. Studies have indicated that fasting may aid in the prevention of health problems such as cancer, diabetes, and Alzheimer's disease.

Intermittent fasting is not as hard as you may think. If anything, it is the exact opposite. There is less planning involved, and many people who have practised it say that they feel more energetic and generally good during the fast. It may be challenging when starting, but the body quickly adapts and you get used to it.

Who Can Fast?

Healthy adults - fasting helps to cleanse the body for any healthy fasting adult.

Children - For children, fasting is only recommended for short periods. Before you get your child to fast, seek your doctor's advice.

People with type 2 diabetes - the effects of type 2 diabetes can be reversed by intermittent fasting. Therefore, if you have this type of diabetes, intermittent fasting is recommended for you.

Who Cannot Fast?

Pregnant women - it is good to keep away from intermittent fasting when pregnant. The body needs more energy and nutrition during pregnancy.

People with any medical conditions - If you have a medical condition related to liver or kidney, fasting is not for you. See your doctor before you start fasting.

People with eating disorders - Fasting is not recommended for persons with eating disorders.

Fasting is optional. If you are afraid of doing it, then don't fast. For positive fasting results, you need not to have fear.

Advantages of Intermittent Fasting
Weight loss

Intermittent fasting alternates between periods of eating and fasting. If you fast, naturally your calorie intake will be reduced. It also helps you maintain your weight loss and prevents you from indulging in mindless eating. Whenever you eat something, your body converts the food into glucose and fat. It uses the glucose immediately and stores the fat for later use. When you skip a few meals, your body starts to reach into its internal stores of fat to provide energy. As soon as the body begins burning fats due to the shortage of glucose, you will start to lose weight. Also, most of the fat that you lose is from the abdominal region. If you want a flat tummy, then this is the perfect diet for you.

Sleep

Lack of sleep is one of the main causes of obesity. When your body doesn't get enough sleep, the internal mechanism of burning fat suffers. Intermittent fasting regulates your sleep cycle, and in turn, makes your body effectively burn fats. A good sleep cycle has different physiological benefits - it makes you feel energetic and elevates your overall mood.

Resistance to illnesses

Intermittent fasting aids in the growth and the regeneration of cells. Did you know that the human body has an internal mechanism that helps repair damaged cells? Intermittent fasting helps kickstart this mechanism. It improves the overall functioning of all the cells in the body. So, it is directly responsible for improving your body's natural defense mechanism by increasing its resistance to diseases and illnesses.

A healthy heart

Intermittent fasting assists in weight loss, and weight loss improves your cardiovascular health. A buildup of plaque in blood vessels is known as atherosclerosis. This is the primary cause for various cardiovascular diseases. The endothelium is the thin lining of blood vessels and any dysfunction in it results in atherosclerosis. Obesity is the primary problem that plagues humanity and is also the main reason for the increase of plaque deposits in the blood vessels. Stress and inflammation also increase the severity of this problem. Intermittent fasting tackles the buildup of fat and helps tackle obesity. So, all you need to do is follow the simple protocols of intermittent fasting to improve your overall health.

A healthy gut

There are several millions of microorganisms present in your digestive system. These microorganisms help improve the overall functioning of your digestive system and are known as the gut microbiome. Intermittent fasting improves the health of this microbiome and improves your digestive health. A healthy digestive system aids in better absorption of food and improves the functioning of your stomach.

Tackles diabetes

Diabetes is a big threat on its own. It is also a primary indicator of the increase in risk factors of various cardiovascular diseases like heart attacks and strokes. When the glucose level increases alarmingly in the bloodstream and there isn't enough insulin to process this glucose, it causes diabetes. When your body resists insulin, it becomes difficult to regulate the insulin levels in the body. Intermittent fasting reduces insulin sensitivity and helps tackle diabetes.

Reduces inflammation

Whenever your body feels there is an internal problem, its natural defense is inflammation. It doesn't mean that all forms of inflammation are desirable. Inflammation can cause several serious health conditions like arthritis, atherosclerosis, and other neurodegenerative disorders.

Any inflammation of this nature is known as chronic inflammation and is quite painful. Chronic inflammation can restrict your body's movements as well. If you want to keep inflammation in check, then intermittent fasting will certainly come in handy.

Promotes cell repair

When you fast, the cells in your body start the process of waste removal. Waste removal means the breaking down of all dysfunctional cells and proteins and is known as autophagy. Autophagy offers protection against several degenerative diseases like Alzheimer's and cancer. You don't like accumulating garbage in your home, do you? Similarly, your body must not hold onto any unnecessary toxins. Autophagy is the body's way of getting rid of all things unnecessary.

Types of Intermittent Fasting

Lean-gains method

The lean-gains method essentially focuses on the combined efforts of rigorous exercise, fasting, and a healthy diet. The fame surrounding this approach comes from its acclaimed success at turning fat directly into muscle. The goal is to fast within each day for 14-16 hours, starting when you wake up.

The ideal approach to lean-gains seems to be that you wake up and fast until 1 pm, doing some stretches and pre-workout warmups just before noon. Starting at noon, you would engage in training in whatever exercise you choose for an hour or less, ending with you breaking your fast around 1 pm. Your meal at this time would be the largest of the day.

You would engage in your day as normal past then, eating again around 4 pm, then eating for the final time around 9 pm, giving yourself a ~15-hour fast until the next day at 1 pm. If you choose this approach yet feel a bit overwhelmed, you can work up to 15 hours, starting with a 13- or 14-hour fast only for the first week, building up to a 15- or 16-hour fast after that.

16:8 Method

The 16:8 method is one of the most popular methods among intermittent fasters. Essentially, you spend 16 hours within each day fasting, and the other 8 hours are your eating window. Most people try to choose their 8-hour eating window to be the times when they're primarily active. If you're a night person, feel free to make it a little later. Hold off eating during the daytime as much as possible then break your fast around 3 or 4 pm. For morning people, break your fast earlier, say, around 11 am, stopping food consumption by 7 pm.

The 16:8 method is an incredibly flexible method that works for many different kinds of people. It's even flexible once you decide to try a particular fasting to eating window ratio. For example, if you don't seem to be jiving with the 11-7 pm eating window, you can absolutely alter the next day to better suit your needs. Try waiting until later in the day to break your fast! Try what you need to do, as long as you're keeping to that 16:8-hour ratio.

Whereas the lean-gains method technically applies the same hourly ratio, it's much more strict regarding healthy diet and exercise regimen. The 16:8 method does not need any type of exercise booster, but that's up to the practitioner. It is always best to try adding healthy dietary choices to one's intermittent fasting eating schedule, but don't try to restrict too many calories, as it can incorporate to feelings of lightheadedness and low energy. With the 16:8 method, you can eat what you need and swap the hours around as desired.

14:10 Method

Similar to the 16:8 method, the 14:10 method requires fasting and eating in varying degrees within each day. In this case, you would fast for 14 hours and engage in eating for a 10-hour window afterward. This method has the same flexibility as the 16:8 method in terms of what time of day it's arranged around, and how easy it is to troubleshoot. It's additionally flexible in the sense that the eating window is two hours longer, accommodating people with more intense physical routines or daily demands, as well as people who simply need to eat a little later in the day to feel well.

20:4 Method

Whereas the 14:10 method was an easier step down from 16:8 method, the 20:4 method is absolutely an increase in terms of difficulty. It's a more intense method, it requires 20 hours of fasting within each day, with only a 4-hour eating window for the individual to gain all his or her nutrients and energy.

A majority of the people who opt to use this method end up having either one large meal with several snacks or they have two smaller meals with fewer snacks. The 20:4 method is flexible in that sense—whereby the individual chooses how the eating window is divided amongst meals and snacks.

The 20:4 method is tricky, many people instinctually over-eat during the eating window, but that's neither necessary nor is it healthy. People that choose the 20:4 method should try to keep meal portions around the same size that they would normally have been without fasting. Experimenting on how many snacks are needed will be helpful as well with this method.

Many people end up working up to the 20:4 method from other methods, based on what their bodies can handle and what they're ready to attempt. Few start with 20:4, so if it's not working for you right away, please don't be too hard on yourself! Step it back to 16:8 and then see how soon you can get back to where you'd like to be.

The Warrior Method

The warrior method is quite similar to the 20:4 method in that the individual fasts for 20 hours within each day and breaks fast for a 4-hour eating window. The difference is in the outlook and mindset of the practitioner, however. Essentially, the thought process behind the warrior method is that, in ancient times, the hunter coming home from stalking prey or the warrior coming home from battle would really only get one meal each day. One meal would have to provide sustenance for the rest of the day, recuperative energy from the ordeal, and sustainable energy for the future.

Therefore, practitioners of warrior method are encouraged to have one large meal when they break their fast, and that meal should be jam-packed with fats, proteins, and carbs for the rest of the day (and for the days ahead). Just like with the 20:4 method, it can sometimes be too intense for practitioners, and it's very easy to scale this one back in forcefulness by making up a method like 18:6 or 17:7. If it's not working, don't force it to work past two weeks, but do try to make it through a week to see if it's your stubbornness or if it's just a mismatch with the method.

12:12 Method

The 12:12 method is a little easier, along the lines of 14:10, rather than 16:8 or 20:4. Beginners to intermittent fasting would do well to try this one right off the bat. Some people get 12 hours of sleep each night and can easily wake up from the fasting period, ready to engage with the eating window. Many people use this method in their lives without even knowing it.

To go about the 12:12 method in your life, you'll want to be as purposeful about it as you can be. Make sure to be strict about your 12-hour cut-offs. Make sure it's working and feeling good in your body, and then you're invited to take things up a notch and try the 14:10 or maybe your own invention, like 15:11. As always, start with what works and then move up (or down) to what feels right (and even possibly better).

5:2 Method

5:2 method is popular among those who want to take things up a notch generally. Instead of fasting and eating within each day, these individuals take up a practice of fasting two whole days out of the week. The other five days are free to eat, exercise, or diet as desired, but those other two days (which can be consecutive or scattered throughout the week) must be strictly fasting days.

For those fasting days, it's not as if the individual can't eat anything altogether, however. In actuality, one is allowed to consume no more than 500 calories each day for this intermittent fasting method. I suppose these fasting days would be better referred to as "restricted-intake" days, for that is a more accurate description.

The 5:2 method is extremely rewarding, but it is also one of the more difficult ones to attempt. If you're having issues with this method, don't be afraid to experiment the next week with a method like 14:10 or 16:8, where you're fasting and eating within each day. If that works better for you, don't be ashamed to embrace it! However, if you're dedicated to having days "on" and days "off" with fasting and eating, there are other alternatives as well.

Eat-Stop-Eat (24-Hour) Method

The eat-stop-eat, or 24-hour method, is another option for people who want to have days "on" and "off" between fasting and eating. It's a little less intense than the 5:2 method, and it's much more flexible for the person, depending on what he or she needs. For instance, if you need a literal 24-hour fast each week and that's it, you can do that. Meanwhile, if you want a more flexible 5:2 method-type thing to happen, you can work with what you want and create a method surrounding those desires and goals.

The most successful approaches to the eat-stop-eat method have involved more strict dieting (or at the very least, cautious and healthy eating) during the five or six days when the individual engages in the week's free-eating window. For the individual to truly see success with weight loss, there will have to be some caloric restriction (or high nutrition focus) those five or six days too, so that the body will have a version of consistency in health and nutrition content.

On the one or two days each week the individual decides to fast, there can still be highly-restricted caloric intake. As with the 5:2 method, he or she can consume no more than 500 calories worth of food and drink during these fasting days, so that the body can maintain energy flow and more.

If the individual engages in exercise, those workout days should absolutely be reserved for the 5 or 6 free-eating days. The same goes for the 5:2 method. Try not to exercise (at least not excessively) on those days that are chosen for fasting. Your body will not appreciate the added stress when you're taking in so few calories. As always, you can choose to move up from eat-stop-eat to another method if this works easily and you're interested in something more. Furthermore, you can start with a strict 24-hour method and then move up to a more flexible eat-stop-eat approach! Do what feels right and never be afraid to troubleshoot one method for the sake of choosing another.

Alternate-Day Method

The alternate-day method is similar to eat-stop-eat and 5:2 methods because it focuses on individual days "on" and "off" for fasting and eating. The difference for this method, in particular, is that it ends up being at least two days a week fasting, and sometimes, it can be as many as four.

Some people follow very strict approaches to alternate-day method and literally fast every other day, only consuming 500 calories or less on those days designated for fasting. Some people, on the other hand, are much more flexible, and they tend to go for two days eating, one day fasting, two days eating, one day fasting, etc. The alternate-day method is even more flexible than eat-stop-eat in that sense, for it allows the individual to choose how he or she alternates between eating and fasting, based on what works for the body and mind the best.

The alternate-day method is like a step up from eat-stop-eat and 24-hour methods, especially if the individual truly alternates one-day fasting and the next day eating, etc. This more intense style of fasting works particularly well for people who are working on equally intense fitness regimens. People who are eating more calories a day than 2000 (which is true for a lot of bodybuilders and fitness buffs) will have more to gain from the alternate-day method, for you only have to cut back your eating on fasting days to about 25 percent of your standard caloric intake. Therefore, those fasting days can still provide solid nutritional support for fitness experts while helping them sculpt their bodies and maintain a new level of health.

Spontaneous Skipping Method

The alternate-day method and eat-stop-eat method are certainly flexible in their approaches to when the individual fasts and when he or she eats. However, none of those mentioned above plans are quite as flexible as the spontaneous skipping method. The spontaneous skipping method literally only requires that the individual skip meals within each day, whenever desired (and when it's sensed that the body can handle it).

Many people with more sensitive digestive systems or who practice more intense fitness regimens will start their experiences with intermittent fasting through the spontaneous skipping method before moving on to something more intensive. People who have very haphazard daily schedules or people who are around food a lot but forget to eat will benefit from this method, for it works well with chaotic schedules and unplanned energies.

Despite that chaotic and unorganized potential, the spontaneous skipping method can also be more structured and organized, depending on what you make of it! For instance, someone desiring more structure can choose which meal each day they'd like to skip. Let's say they choose to skip breakfast each day. Then, their spontaneous skipping method will be structured around making sure to skip breakfast (a.k.a.—not to eat until at least 12 pm) daily. Whatever you need to do to make this method work, try it! This method is made for experimentation and adventurousness.

Crescendo Method

This method is very well-suited for female practitioners (since their anatomies can be so detrimentally sensitive to high-intensity fasts). Essentially, this approach is made for internal awareness, gentle introductions, and gradual additions, depending on what works and what doesn't. It's a very active, trial-and-error type of method.

Through the crescendo method, the individual starts by only fasting two or three days a week, and on those fast days, it wouldn't be a very intense fast at all. In fact, it wouldn't even be so strict that the individual would have to consume no more than 500 calories, like with 5:2, eat-stop-eat, and other methods. Instead, these "fasting" days would be trial periods for methods like the 12:12, 14:10, 16:8, or 20:4. The remaining four or five days out of the week would be open eating-window periods, but again, the practitioner is encouraged to maintain a healthy diet throughout the week.

The crescendo method works extremely well for female practitioners because it enables them to see how methods like 14:10 or 12:12 will affect their bodies without tying them to the method hook, line, and sinker. It allows them to see what each method does to their hormone levels, their menstruation tendencies, and their mood swings. Therefore, the crescendo method encourages these people to be more in touch with their bodies before moving too quickly into something that could do serious anatomical and hormonal damage.

The crescendo method will work extremely well for overweight or diabetic practitioners too, for it will allow them to have these same "trial period" moments with all the methods before choosing what feels and works best, based on each individual situation.

How Intermittent Fasting Works

There is a lot of science behind why intermittent fasting works. Intermittent fasting works because it restricts the body of toxins and allows itself to clear out any excess. It gives the body a break and provides a moment to recalibrate. With this recalibration, neurotransmitters are released easier in the brain, and one's senses of hunger is adjusted back to how it should be. Once food is eaten after the fast, nutritional absorption is boosted throughout the entire body, to the benefit of all of one's organs.

Additionally, intermittent fasting recalibrates one's hormones in relation to stress and hunger so that balanced mood, patience, and intellect can be increased despite the seeming lack of food. Intermittent fasting tells the brain and body to restart. It makes your system go back to basics and clean out any gunk, and a lot of that gunk tends to be stored fat or water weight. It sees the toxins in your body and refuses to let you hold onto them. Overall, intermittent fasting proves that a change in routine can have great and lasting effects on one's health.

Chapter 2: Foods to Eat/Avoid

It is very important to know the foods which are good for you when starting intermittent fasting. Some other foods may not be good for you.

Foods to Eat

You will definitely need to consume energy giving foods when fasting. These foods give you energy that is enough to sustain your body until the next meal. The following foods are good for you:

- Cruciferous vegetables like cauliflower, brussel sprouts, broccoli, and more are full of fiber and so much more!
- Avocado is high in healthy fats and calories, so it's perfect to have as a snack or in a meal.
- Potatoes of all kinds are great to satisfy one's hunger and provide a nutritional punch.
- Legumes and beans of all varieties contain good carbohydrates that can help lower weight without too much restriction of calories.
- Berries contain vitamin C, flavonoids, and antioxidants that will add a lot of good to your fast.
- Eggs of any animal are packed with protein to help you build muscle and retain energy during the fast.
- Wild-caught fish have a great amount of protein as well as vitamin D for one's brain and healthy fats and omega-3s for one's body.
- Anything high in protein or high in probiotic content will be good to have along for the ride.
- Grains and nuts are full of fiber, and healthy fats for snacks or meals during your fast's eating windows.

- Spices such as cayenne pepper, psyllium husk, or dried dandelion are natural weight loss agents that can help anyone's process.

Foods to Avoid

- Sugary foods may curb your appetite, but they won't do anything good for your body in the long run. Steer clear for your future ease.
- Processed foods will be the most important things to avoid, especially as you prepare for your fast.
- Highly GMO foods are also things to avoid when you're working through your fast. They can offset the actual nutrition being provided by other foods in your diet.

Drinks to Take

You are allowed to take drinks while fasting. Go for drinks that are nutritious because they are good for the body. Some of the drinks that you can take are listed below:

I. Water with fruit or veggie slices will provide nourishment and flavor for those times when you're fasting and need a little extra boost!

II. Probiotic drinks like kombucha or kefir will work to heal your gut and tide you over till the next eating window.

III. Black coffee will become your new best friend but be sure not to add cream and sugar! They detract from the good work coffee can do for your body during intermittent fasting.

IV. Teas of any kind are soothing as well as healing for various elements of the body, mind, and soul. Once again, be sure to omit the cream and sugar!

V. Chilled or heated broths made from vegetables, bone, or animals can sustain one's energy during times of fast, too.

VI.   Apple cider vinegar shots are great for the tummy and for healing overall! Hippocrates' remedy for any ailment included this and a healthy regimen of fasting occasionally, so you're sure to succeed with this trick.

VII.   Water with salt can provide electrolytes, hydration, and brief sustenance for anyone whose stomachs won't stop grumbling.

VIII.   Fresh-pressed juices are always great for the body, mind, and soul, and in times of intermittent fasting, they can sustain one's energy and mood during day-long fast periods, in particular.

IX.   Wheatgrass shots are just as healthy as ACV shots, with a whole other subset of benefits. To awaken your body and give a jolt to your system, try these on for size.

X.   Coconut water is more hydrating than standard water, and it's full of additional nutrients, too! Try this alternative if you need some enhancement to your usual water.

Drinks to Keep Off

I.   Sodas of any kind, whether diet or non-diet, are to be avoided absolutely. They are high in sugar and riddled with terrible things for your body. Try to steer clear of this drink, especially during fasting periods.

II.   Coconut and almond drinks that are high in sugar are also to be avoided. Artificial sweeteners are killers for one's blood sugar and insulin levels. They will reverse all the good work you've done, so be cautious.

III.   Alcohol will distract you from your focus and commitment to the fast. It will also steer your body off-course from where you want it to be. Try to intermittent fast soberly.

Chapter 3: Myths About Intermittent Fasting

There are many myths out there about intermittent fasting. Some of the common ones are as follows:

MYTH: Your body will definitely enter into starvation mode.

TRUTH: Your body will definitely not enter into starvation mode through intermittent fasting. Skipping meals or adjusting to longer periods between meals where you don't eat is not going to make you starve. It's going to help your body remember how to absorb nutrients and you will thrive instead.

MYTH: You'll lose muscle in this endeavor.

TRUTH: This myth goes along the same lines as the first one above. Just like your body won't enter into starvation mode (unless something goes very, very wrong or you're trying to do too much); your body won't lose muscle through intermittent fasting. The only reason why intermittent fasting would cause muscle loss would be if it was causing you to starve, but once again, the first myth addresses this falsity, making this myth false as well.

MYTH: You'll almost assuredly overeat during eating windows, and that's not healthy at all.

TRUTH: While some people will have the instinct to overeat during eating windows, not everyone will overeat. Even those who do at the start will realize how to move forward without this overeating instinct in the future. Your body will urge you to overeat because, at the start, it won't realize what you're doing to it, but as long as you keep portion sizes largely the same and don't gorge on snacks, your body will adjust and so will your appetite.

MYTH: Your metabolism will slow down dangerously.

TRUTH: People who think this myth is true, only assume that restricted caloric intake will make one's metabolism slow down over time, but these individuals forget that intermittent fasting isn't necessarily about cutting down calories overall (although methods like 20:4 don't leave much room for full caloric intake). It's actually about cutting down the times during which one consumes calories. There needn't be any caloric restriction whatsoever! It just depends on the practitioner and what he or she decides to do with dieting in addition to intermittent fasting.

MYTH: You'll only gain weight if you try skipping meals.

TRUTH: This myth is based on the same logic that drives the myth about overeating. If you gorge yourself during your eating windows, you'll surely gain weight, but hardly anyone will continuously gorge with intermittent fasting. Anyone who tries will realize how unsuccessful it is, so he or she will not continuously gorge in response. Anyone who doesn't realize his or her efforts with eating are unsuccessful will soon realize that something's wrong, as his or her weight shows no improvement. Skipping meals never necessarily means that someone will gain weight. It just means that people who skip meals and gorge or overeat when it is mealtime won't see the desired effects.

MYTH: During fasting periods, you literally can't eat anything.

TRUTH: This myth is partially true and partially false. It's true only for methods like 12:12, 14:10, 16:8, and 20:4 that require fasting and eating in alternation within each individual day. For the 12:12 method, for example, you'd spend 12 hours fasting and

12 hours eating. In this case, you would definitely not eat anything or consume any calories during that 12-hour fasting window, but the same isn't true for methods that alternate between days "on" and days "off" between fasting and eating. For those types of methods, you absolutely can eat during fasting periods! It might feel counterintuitive as you read these words, but you don't explicitly have to eat nothing during fast periods. Most methods that have full days of fasting actually allow for caloric intake as long as it's restricted by 20-25 percent of one's normal intake. Therefore, for methods like 5:2, alternate-day, eat-stop-eat, and crescendo, on days when you're fasting, you can still consume around 500 calories, and that will help a lot!

MYTH: There's only one way to do intermittent fasting that's right and truly the best.

TRUTH: This myth is absolutely and utterly false. There is no one right way to practice intermittent fasting, and part of the beauty of intermittent fasting is that there are so many different methods, meaning each approach to intermittent fasting, likely has a few different options to choose from. Similarly, different body and personality types will be drawn to different methods, based on individuals' abilities and goals. Intermittent fasting is about flexibility, adjustment, and self-correction. There's no one right method for everyone, and there's no "best" method to strive for. Do whatever method feels right and suits your life, and once you've found it, practice it as long as you can! That's far more realistic and accessible.

MYTH: It's not natural to fast like that.

TRUTH: It's more natural to practice intermittent fasting then it is to eat three full meals each day! It's more connected to our evolutionary drives and to our primitive selves to eat like this.

It's better for our brains, hearts, cells, and digestive systems to have a break from food once in a while to recalibrate. As you learned in the Introduction, people have been practicing intermittent fasting for as long as humans have been in existence. It's only myths like this that circulate today that make it seem like intermittent fasting is foreign, unhealthy, and dangerous. Animals of all types become healthier after periods of fasting, and humans are no different. Remember that we are animals and that intermittent fasting is in our nature. Proceed with that confidence and knowledge!

Chapter 4: Mistakes to Avoid While on Intermittent Fasting

Now that you are aware of the protocols of intermittent fasting and the benefits it offers, you must be quite excited to get started! Before you start this diet, you need to be aware of a couple of common mistakes that you need to avoid. If you avoid the mistakes discussed in this chapter, then you can maximize the benefits you derive from this diet.

1. Giving up too soon

Intermittent fasting might not be easy during the initial weeks. You will need to go for prolonged periods of time without eating. Whichever method you choose, discipline is of importance to ensure that you stick to your diet. During the initial week or two, you will need to combat your hunger pangs if you want this diet to be successful. If you can manage it for about seven days or so, you will start to see the positive benefits of this diet. Therefore, you should not give up too soon. Instead, trust the process and the diet and you will see positive results within no time.

2. Binge eating

When you break your fast, you might be tempted to stuff yourself with a lot of food. If you start overloading on calories after fasting for 16 hours, it will negate the benefits of this diet. If you indulge in binge eating whenever you break your fast, this diet will not do you any good. Instead, pace yourself and eat slowly. Your stomach takes about twenty minutes to realize when you are feeling full. So, take your time while eating and don't eat if you aren't hungry.

3. Not eating enough

You need to eat until you are full and no more than that. If you don't eat anything at all, then you run the risk of starving yourself. If your body shifts into starvation mode, then you cannot achieve your weight loss and health goals. A lot of people worry that they will undo all that they have achieved while fasting if they eat during the eating window. If you do this, it will be quite difficult to go through the subsequent spell of fasting. Your body needs food to function optimally. So, if you skip meals unnecessarily or if you don't eat enough food, you are merely hurting yourself.

4. Wrong foods

You need to eat the right foods if you want to lose weight or achieve your fitness goals on this diet. It isn't merely about the calories you consume, but about the quality of nutrition, you feed your body. If you fast for 12 hours and then eat a tub of ice cream, it certainly will not do you any good! The way your body metabolizes food is quite different. For instance, if you consume 500-calories of avocado it will be metabolized quite differently from 500 calories of cookies or chips! Also, if you end up eating junk food after breaking your fast, it is quite likely that you will be hungry within no time at all.

The protocols of Intermittent Fasting dictate that you need to eat a healthy and a well-balanced meal after breaking your fast! Ensure that you consume the necessary macros before you think about indulging in any junk food. Fill yourself up with protein and fiber-rich food, healthy dietary fats, and some carbs before you even think about reaching for a chocolate bar.

5. Forgetting to drink

You need to consume calorie-free beverages throughout the day to keep your body thoroughly hydrated. If you don't drink plenty of water and stay thirsty for long periods, it can trigger unnecessary hunger pangs. Usually, hunger pangs are a sign that your body is thirsty. Also, if you keep your body hydrated, you will feel satiated while fasting.

6. Taking it too far

Occasionally, you might not be able to fast for 16 hours at a stretch and you might want to break your fast earlier than usual. If that's the case, then please do so, but don't make a habit of it. Listening to your body is necessary. Your body knows what it needs. Intermittent fasting isn't about numbers. Instead, it is about doing what is good for your body. Don't take it too far and risk burning yourself out.

If you avoid the common mistakes discussed in this chapter, it will be quite easy to stick to intermittent fasting.

Chapter 5: Tips and Tricks for a Successful Intermittent Fasting
Your mind is the most significant hurdle

Implementing intermittent fasting is easy. When you eat depends on the form of intermittent fasting you decide to follow. If you want to fast daily, then it can be something as simple as giving your breakfast a miss when you wake up. Instead, you start your eating window with lunch and go about your day as usual. However, there is a mental barrier that you might come across. You might wonder how you can go through your day without breakfast. Do you feel that you will faint if you don't eat or that you will not be able to think straight? These questions are natural, and it is okay if you have any reservations about this diet. When you try this diet, you will understand that all these fears are unwarranted. Nothing will happen to your body if you don't eat one meal a day. In fact, you will feel better and more energetic than you ever did. If you keep thinking that you need to eat every couple of hours or have five meals daily or have your breakfast, or whatever it is that you have convinced yourself of, it is all in your mind. You believe all this because you were told it, not because you ever tried it for yourself. Your ability to think is essential. If you can think differently, you can act differently as well.

It is easy to lose weight

When you tend to eat less frequently, your overall food intake reduces. As a result of all this, you will end up losing weight while you follow intermittent fasting. You might plan for big meals but eating them consistently will not be easy. Intermittent fasting is an excellent idea for all those who want to lose weight because it merely reduces your overall carb intake. Even if you have two large meals daily, the calories you eat will undoubtedly be less than when you ate six meals a day. By merely cutting down on how much you eat, you can lose weight. After all, it is quite simple to lose weight. So, if weight loss is your primary aim, then you accomplish it with this simple diet.

If you want, you can build muscle

You can build muscle while you fast. You shouldn't worry about losing muscle while on this diet. Also, the muscle you gain will be lean muscle. If you want to have a lean and toned body, then this is the best diet for you.

You can work while you fast

You will realize that you are more productive while you're on a fast. Your energy levels will be quite high when you wake up in the morning. The first three hours of the morning will be the most productive portion of the day for you. Well, that's about 12 to 15 hours into your diet, and that's when your body functions optimally. You might believe that your brain will not function optimally when it doesn't get the necessary glucose. Well, all that's just a misconception. Since you do not need to worry about what you can eat for breakfast, you can use this time to do something that's more productive. Your body produces energy while you sleep, and you can utilize this store of power as soon as you wake up. If you want to become productive, then you certainly must give this diet a go.

Cycle what you eat

Intermittent fasting works well. However, calorie and carb cycling can make it more efficient. Do you know what these terms mean? You must have a couple of extra calories on the day you decide to exercise. So, you cycle calories by increasing your food intake. On the other days, you must aim for a calorie deficit. The idea behind this logic is quite simple. You can train to build muscle on all those days you exercise and, on the other days, you can encourage your body to burn fat. You must cycle your carbs on the day you train. It helps to stimulate the loss of fat. Have high protein and low-fat meals on regular days and the days you work out, have some carbs.

It is a lifestyle

We often tend to think of our diets as short-term regimes. It is better to be mindful of what you eat throughout the week instead of just a day or a couple of hours. Whether you have a protein shake 30 minutes before you work out isn't much of an issue if you have a high protein meal within 24-hours of your workout. Intermittent fasting works because of the eating restriction it places on you. Let us say that you have three meals daily; it is a grand total of 21 meals in a week. Over the course of the diet, do you think your body cares if you eat from 8 a.m. to 8 p.m. in the day or from 1 p.m. to 1 a.m.? How about we stretch it out for a month. Would it make sense to have 80 well-balanced meals so that your body can make the most of it regardless of the time frame within which you eat?

It is essential to understand that the food you eat usually has a great impact on your overall health. The diet will not make any sense if you starve yourself daily and then break your fast with all sorts of junk. It is better to think of Intermittent Fasting as a lifestyle choice instead of a mere diet. Not only does it make the diet more practical to follow, but you can maintain your weight loss as well. If you follow the diet religiously for two months and then go back to your unhealthy ways, it will not do your body any good. In fact, all the good that the diet did will be nullified.

You will want less food

When you fast, you will realize that your body craves less food. The diet doesn't victimize you. In fact, it teaches you to listen to your body. You will do what your body tells you to. While you fast, you might think of a hundred different things you want to eat, but when you break your fast, your opinion is bound to change. Once you get used to the diet, you will want to eat only when you are hungry. In a way, intermittent fasting curbs mindless eating.

Lose fat and gain muscle

If you want to lose fat and build lean muscle, then you must follow Intermittent Fasting, carb cycling, and calorie cycling. It is not practically possible to lose gain muscle and even lose fat simultaneously. To lose weight, your body needs to burn more calories than you consume. So, it is essential to maintain a net calorie deficit to shed weight. However, if you want to build muscle, you need to consume more calories than you burn. It is apparent that you cannot have a net surplus and a net deficit simultaneously. For instance, you can either eat more than 2000 calories or less than 2000 calories at a given point in time. It is the reason why it is impossible to burn excess fat and gain muscle at the same time. However, if you don't think about the small timeframe and think about the diet over the course of a month instead of a day, you have more options available. For instance, you can decide to work out three days a week, and you can maintain a calorie deficit on all the other days of the week. Therefore, your body will lose fat on a couple of days and gain muscle on the rest. But you cannot do both at the same time. So, you must think about your diet from a long-term perspective instead of a day-to-day diet.

More gains when you fast

There is a simple hypothesis for strength training, and it goes as follows "Always do the most important thing before the rest." It is about prioritizing. It works well not just for your diet, but with any other aspect of your life as well. It is quite simple. You must set one goal for your workout schedule, and you must do the exercises that are more important than others. For instance, let us assume that you work out three days in a week - Monday, Wednesday and Friday. You can do two sessions every session, the upper body workout, and the lower body workout. The results you derive from exercise are more when you are fasting.

Fasted state

If you don't exceed 50 calories, your body will stay in a fasted state. There is no scientific evidence about whether it is true or not, but it seems to work for the majority. So, if you like to start your day with a glass of orange juice or a cup of coffee, then you can do so without any worry. Just make sure that your calorie intake doesn't exceed 50 calories. The idea of an intermittent fast is to switch your body to a fasted state instead of a fed state. It is quite easy, and you don't have to make any drastic changes to your daily schedule.

Drink lots of water

You must prepare yourself to drink plenty of water while you fast. Most of us aren't used to drinking a lot of water. In fact, we tend to forget that our body needs water. You can rectify this situation by drinking water. You must have at least eight glasses of water daily, and intermittent fasting will help you. Drinking plenty of water helps to detoxify your body and improves the health of your skin as well.

The best diet

Who would not want the ultimate diet plan? Everyone wants one. However, there is no such thing as a perfect diet. The diet that works well for one person might not work for someone else. Some might prefer the 24-hour method and others might like Lean gains. The idea is to follow a diet that works well for you. If you want, you can try the different variations of intermittent fasting before you select one method. Your body isn't the same as someone else's, and its metabolism differs as well.

It is essential to stay motivated even when you don't seem to lose any weight while on an intermittent fast. So, you successfully made it through the first week or two of intermittent fasting, but you don't notice any weight loss? You will probably not see any fat loss within the first two weeks of the diet, which is normal. Fat loss starts only after three weeks of the diet. So, you need to keep going even when you feel like it's not working. Maybe you are in a slump and cannot see the results that you once could. It is important that you don't lose faith in the diet and that you keep going even when you don't want to. All that sounds simple, but how can you stay motivated?

While you follow intermittent fasting, you will feel quite energetic and sharp when you wake up in the morning. In fact, you will feel more energetic than ever. Your body will start to function optimally. The best part about this diet is that you can do everything like you normally would. Concentrate on how good you felt while on this diet, and it will motivate you. A little bit of self-control and self-discipline can help you stay on track. If you feel that a method isn't working for you, try another method and see if that works. Try different foods. It is a trial and error process. So, don't give up just yet.

Chapter 6: Eating Out

In this chapter, you will learn about a couple of different strategies that you can follow while eating out.

Nutrition Plan

Track your nutritional intake while at home. You must be aware of the number of calories that you consume, the size of the portions, and the composition of your meals. For instance, if you consume 1800 calories in three meals, your dinner can make up for 700 calories, lunch for 400 calories and the rest for another meal. It means that you can have about 70g of protein for lunch and dinner and about 40g in another meal.

Stick to the Same Foods

Once you establish your calculated nutrition plan, it is all about sticking to it as much as you can while eating out. Ideally, you must try to stick to similar foods to those that you eat while at home. For instance, if you are used to a meal of meats and vegetables, then order something similar when you go out for a meal. If you go out for a meal, stick to the protein and fibers you eat at home and skip any carb and sugar-rich foods.

Increase Protein

Once you establish your calculated nutrition plan, it is all about sticking to it as much as you can while eating out. Ideally, you must try to stick to similar foods to those that you eat while at home. For instance, if you are used to a meal of meats and vegetables, then order something similar when you go out for a meal. If you go out for a meal, stick to the protein and fibers you eat at home and skip any carb and sugar-rich foods.

Carbs

You need to be careful about the number of carbs you consume. If the dish you ordered has more carbohydrates than you are used to consuming, then simply skip the carbs. You need to avoid carbs as much as possible if you want to speed up the process of weight loss. Carbs will fill you up for a while and then you will feel hungry again. Instead, fill up on the foods that are good for you. If there is a bread basket on the table, please resist the urge of reaching for it.

Post Meal Hunger

If you want to have a dessert or still have the urge to eat more, even though you are aware that it will exceed your ideal calorie intake, then you need to know that this feeling of hunger will subside soon. A simple trick is to have a cup of tea after a meal, it will make you feel full. You can also go for a walk after eating, and you will feel full. It takes about 20 minutes for your brain to signal to you that you are full, so don't keep stuffing yourself with food.

If you follow these simple steps, you can stick to your diet even when you go out for a meal.

Chapter 7: Scientific Facts About Intermittent Fasting

Intermittent fasting has been found to help people lose weight and also promote their health. However, conventional calorie restrictions diets are superior to intermittent fasting. This is according to a study called HELENA- Intermittent fasting's largest research in history. It was done by scientists from Heidelberg University Hospital and the German Cancer Research Center (DKFZ). They found out that there are different routes to achieve a healthier weight. You just have to get a diet plan that suits you best.

Increased Brain Cell Production

This is one of the most surprising yet amazing benefits of intermittent fasting. Fasting has been shown to enhance neurogenesis, which is the process of developing new brain cells and nerves. Optimizing the brain's neurogenesis can help to improve your mood, focus, memory, and other cognitive functions.

In fact, one study published in the Journal of *Cerebral Blood Flood and Metabolism* shows that mice that fasted produced more brain cells than mice on a regular diet. The researchers measured cell production, cell death, and neurogenesis. Following three months of intermittent fasting, the mice that fasted showed an increase in brain cells and had less brain cell damage from a stroke.

Another study, *Chronic Intermittent Fasting Improves Cognitive Functions and Brain Structures in Mice*, by Liaoliao Li, Zhi Wang, and Zhiyi Zuo , showed that intermittent fasting leads to improvements in cognitive functions and brain activity in mice. Seven week old mice were either put on an alternate-day fasting or a high-fat diet for 11 months. There was a substantial difference between the two groups. Mice on the alternate day fasting diet had higher levels of learning and memory, more cell production in the brain, and lower levels of oxidative stress. In comparison, mice on the high-fat diet were obese with hyperlipidemia and had poor exercise tolerance and performance.

Research shows that fasting may have a similar positive effect on your brain as exercise has on your body. Both of these activities place stress on the brain, making it stronger and more resistant to stressful stimuli. The brain reacts to stressful stimuli by building up new neurons and connections.

Both exercise and fasting seem to boost ketones and mitochondria production within the brain. In addition, new neural connections and synapses are created and strengthened. This leads to better memory and learning.

Increased BDNF production

Besides promoting neurogenesis, fasting increases brain-derived neurotrophic factor (BDNF). BDNF is a growth factor and is critical for cognitive function. BDNF produces new brain cells and nerves and creates connections between them. It also helps with learning and memory and is a natural antidepressant. Higher levels of BDNF keeps neurons healthy and ensures the neurons communicate effectively with one another. In contrast, lower levels of BDNF can increase the risks of memory loss, dementia, and other cognitive problems.

According to a study by Bronwen Martin, Mark P. Mattson, and Stuart Maudsley (2006), fasting for 16 to 18 hours can increase BDNF production by as much as 100 percent, and fasting for 36 hours can increase BDNF production by as much 400 percent.

Other research by the National Institute on Aging in the U.S. has shown that mice who fasted every other day showed improvements in their cognitive functioning. The team of researchers put 40 mice on an alternate day fasting schedule (one day on, one day off) and noted that the parts of their brain responsible for memory were more active.

In addition, the brain protein, brain-derived neurotrophic factor (BDNF), increased by up to 50 percent in the mice that fasted.

May protect against Alzheimer's

Alzheimer's is a type of dementia that gradually destroys memory and mental function over time. Currently, there isn't a cure for Alzheimer's. One study looked at whether intermittent fasting improved the cognitive function of people with Alzheimer's. Researchers looked at ten people with early signs of Alzheimer's. Each person was asked to make a number of lifestyle modifications, including fasting for 12 hours each night. Six months later, Nine out of the ten subjects showed improvements in their cognitive abilities.

How Intermittent Fasting Impacts HGH

When you fast, your HGH increase. This helps to preserve lean muscle and breaks down fat. When free fatty acids are released and converted into energy, this process is known as lipolysis. Obese individuals generally have inefficient lipolysis processes. Lower HGH levels may be one possible cause of this.

Besides fasting, HGH levels can also be increased by exercise. These levels can fluctuate throughout the day since the pituitary gland releases HGH hormone in spurts. Our HGH levels are generally higher when we wake up. We produce growth hormone during sleep, which increases our blood glucose that can be used as fuel for the day. Thus, this idea that you have to eat breakfast to get energy is false. Your body is already primed and ready to function in the morning without having to load up on food.

In addition, many popular breakfast choices, such as cereals and toasts, are high in sugar and carbs. This can make you feel lethargic and tired.

HGH is a natural testosterone booster and has been shown to increase muscle strength and improve exercise performance. In fact, many bodybuilders and athletes may inject additional HGH to improve their performance. A study by the International Journal of Endocrinology, looked at the effects of HGH on muscle strength in men over 50-years-old. Fourteen healthy male subjects were divided into two groups: seven subjects were placed in the HGH therapy group, while the remaining seven were placed in the placebo group. Six months later, all the participants were tested for their body composition and muscle strength, including a number of exercises, such as the leg press and bench press exercises. The HGH group showed a significant increase in muscle strength in the lower body compared to the placebo group.

One study by the Journal of Clinical Investigation showed that intermittent fasting dramatically increased the growth hormone production in men.

Another study from the Journal of Clinical Endocrinology and Metabolism showed that intermittent fasting reduced leptin levels in obese adults. This led to instantaneous increases in testosterone levels.

A fascinating study by the European Journal of Endocrinology showed that fasting dramatically increased the Gonadotropin-

Releasing Hormone (GnRH), a testosterone precursor, in both obese and non-obese men. The researchers looked at 17 men who were divided into two groups (Nine men in the obese group and eight men in the non-obese group). GnRH levels in the obese men rose by 26 percent while the GnRH levels in non-obese men rose by 67 percent. In addition, serum testosterone levels shot up by 180 percent in those in the non-obese group.

Fasting and Leptin

Fasting is one way to increase leptin and glucose sensitivity. Leptin levels have been shown to fall after a short-term fast and return back to normal after eating. Any forms of fasting should work since it forces the body to burn through excess glucose stores.

One study published in the Journal of Clinical Endocrinology & Metabolism looked at how fasting affected leptin levels in nine obese men. After three days of fasting, the researchers noted that the subjects had reductions in total body mass (21.4 ± 3.7%) and leptin (76.3 ± 8.1%). Leptin levels returned to baseline levels within 12 hours of eating.

Another study published in Metabolism looked at the changes in serum leptin and endocrine in both men and women after 7 days of fasting. The subjects were made up of 11 men and 13 women. After 7 days of fasting, the researchers noted that both men and women lost an average of 4 percent in body weight. Leptin decreased in both men (from 3.7 ± 0.5 to 2.1 ± 0.4 ng/mL) and women (16.2 ± 1.9 ng/mL to 6.0 ± 0.8 ng/mL) following fasting. Compared to men, women had higher levels of leptin before and after calorie restriction. However, women showed a bigger decrease in leptin levels overall.

As these studies show, fasting seems to be effective at reducing leptin levels and body mass in both men and women.

Fasting and Inflammation?

There is evidence that intermittent fasting may be an effective way to reduce inflammation. Research shows that intermittent fasting may have a protective effect against high blood pressure, high insulin, and inflammation. There is also evidence that shows fasting may help with type 2 diabetes and autoimmune conditions like MS and rheumatoid arthritis.

In a study published by National Center for Biotechnology Information, researchers fed mice either a low-fat or high-fat diet for 10-12 weeks. After fasting, the mice were fed a low-fat diet and lost more body weight (18% compared to 5%), performed better on memory and learning tasks, and showed better locomotor activity compared to the mice on a high-fat diet. Low-fat mice also had an improved nervous system and immune function. The researchers concluded that fasting has an anti-inflammatory effect on the neuroimmune system, which a high-fat diet prevents.

Ramadan fasting has been shown to have a positive effect on reducing inflammation and may even help to treat fatty liver. One study published in the US National Library of Medicine in 2017, compared 83 people with non-alcoholic fatty liver disease (NAFLD), 42 who fasted and 41 controls who didn't fast for Ramadan. Those who fasted showed significant reductions in glucose, plasma insulin, insulin resistance, and inflammation compared to the non-fasting group.

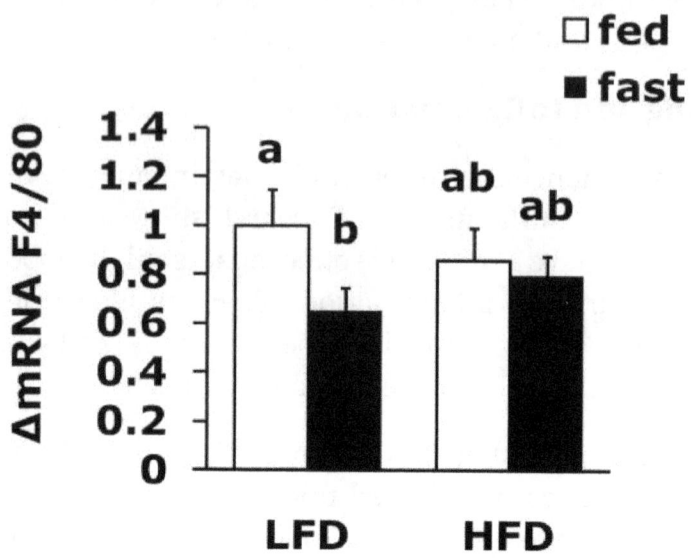

A. Fasting reduces expression of brain F4/80

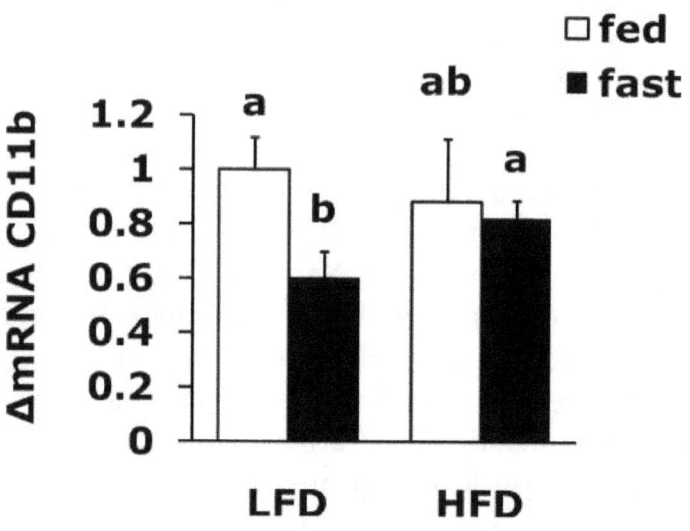

B. Fasting reduces expression of brain CD11b

Fasting reduces expression of brain F4/80 and CD11b which an HFD diet prevents

Fasting lowers expression of brain CD11b and F4/80 which a high-fat diet (HFD) diet prevents. Mice were fed either a high fat diet (HFD) or low-fat diet (LFD) for 12 weeks. Then, the mice were fasted (fast) or fed for 24 hours. (a) Quantitative PCR (qPCR) was used to quantify F4/80 mRNA from whole brain. Results are expressed as relative fold change in mRNA expression (ΔmRNA), means ± s.e.m.; n = 8; main effect of state (P = 0.003). (b) qPCR was used to quantify CD11b mRNA from brain. Results are expressed as relative fold change in mRNA expression (ΔmRNA), means ± s.e.m.; n = 8; main effect of state (P = 0.004). Bars without a common superscript letter are different (P < 0.05).

28-Day Diet Plan

The fasting for this 28-Day plan is based on 14-10 type. With this type, you will have early supper so as to make sure that you fast for 10 hours.

The Shopping List
Day 1-7

5 oz Butter	14oz Dates
13oz Bacon	15oz honey
5oz baby Spinach	16 Pork
16Eggs	12oz Dark molasses
5 oz Heavy cream	14oz Orange juice
20oz Cheese	10oz Curry powder
17oz Salt	17oz Cauliflower rice
10oz Pepper	16oz Lettuce leaves
10 Chicken breasts	10oz Sour cream
15 Garlic cloves	16oz Olive oil
5 Ginger	16oz Black pepper
5oz Tamarind	16 oz Rosemary
400ml Soy sauce	5 Egg whites
400g Basil Leaves	10oz Cooking spray
10oz Lime juice	10ozSmoked paprika
250g Palm sugar	12oz Tomato paste
24oz Fish sauce	14oz Apple cider vinegar
3 Red chilis	24oz Tomatoes
8oz Rice noodles	10oz Bone broth
5oz carrots	10oz Chili powder
10oz Onions	4 Lemons
5oz Coriander	16oz Salmon fillets
5oz Roasted peanuts	12oz Cream cheese
12oz Mint leaves	15oz Capers
1oz Salmon	2 Avocados
30oz Ghee	17 oz Blueberries
15oz Lemon juice	¼ liter Coconut milk
5oz Psyllium Husk Powder	24oz Kales
	20oz Turkey
15oz Coconut oil	10oz Chives

-46-

12oz Berries	8oz Maple flavored syrup
10oz Italian seasoning	20oz Asparagus
8oz Balsamic vinegar	12oz Baking powder
4oz Bacon	15oz Whole wheat flour
5oz Mushroom	8oz Flour
8oz Fresh thyme	12oz Vanilla
15oz Salad dressing	21g Milk
10oz Almonds	12oz Spaghetti squash
10oz Chia seeds	3 Yellow peppers
10oz flax seeds	17oz Beef Steak
15oz Peanut butter	10oz Whipping cream
10oz Hemp seeds	12oz Celery stalks
8oz Oats	10oz Mayo
24oz Greek yogurt	12oz Brown mustard
1-liter Canola oil	8oz Dill
20oz Beets	8oz Pecans
8oz Garlic powder	12oz Coconut aminos
8oz Onion powder	
15oz Sweet potato	

Day 8-14

2 packets Whole wheat flour	12oz Applesauce
10oz Cooking spray	10oz Cinnamon
16oz Walnuts	1 packet All-purpose flour
2 Apples	14oz Mayonnaise
17oz Almond milk	10oz Baking soda
12oz Honey	12oz Raw almonds
18oz Bacon	14ozTart cherries
16oz Ghee	16oz Vanilla
20 Garlic cloves	8oz Maple syrup
17oz Salt	10oz Greek yogurt
12 Onions	8oz Fennel bulb
12oz Black pepper	12oz Parsley sprigs
24oz Potatoes	12oz Manzanilla sherry
14oz Brussels sprout	10oz Raw prawns

1oz Olive oil	10oz Tomato paste
8oz Red vinegar	1 Bread
14oz Pepper	10oz Dill
10oz Thyme	8oz Cayenne pepper
8oz cumin	12oz Almond flour
1 Challah bread	14oz Dairy-free milk
8 eggs	9ozMaple syrup
10oz Vanilla extract	8oz Chia seeds
34oz Sugar	14.5oz Coconut flour
20oz Butter	8oz Shrimp
18oz Rum	8oz Arrowroot powder
5 Bananas	11oz Sriracha
2 24 oz. canned rinsed baked beans	8oz Ketchup
16oz Vegetable stock	18oz Lamb
10 Tomatoes	2 Lemons
12oz Basil	12oz Extra virgin oil
6 Lemons	10oz Dried oregano
10oz Okra	12oz Blackberries
17oz Cassava flour	5 Bananas
18oz Coconut oil	12oz Raspberries
10oz Baking powder	12oz Blueberries
16oz Buttermilk	18oz Milk
1 Pineapple	16oz Plain yogurt
10oz Maraschino cherries	10oz Fish
11oz Cauliflower	10oz Cucumber
12oz Garlic powder	14oz Cherry tomatoes
6 Carrots	12oz Black olives
16oz Coconut aminos	8oz Crab legs
2 Sweet potatoes	8 Pork sausages
10oz Paprika	8oz Mushroom
8oz Avocado oil	10oz Parsley
16oz Lemon juice	1 Whole chicken
	1 Lamb rack
	6oz Rosemary

Day 15-21

11 Eggs	24oz Prosciutto de parma
10oz oats	16oz Cod fillets
12oz Cinnamon	12oz Capers
16oz Low-fat cottage cheese	10oz Avocado oil
1 Pineapple	12oz Almond flour
16 oz Pork tenderloin	10oz Erythritol
12oz Onion	6 lemons
8oz Tapioca starch	6oz Balsamic vinegar
8oz Ginger	6oz Honey
12 oz Pineapple juice	12oz Green plantains
8oz Bell paper	16oz Greek yogurt
6oz Coconut aminos	6oz Coconut butter
8oz Garlic cloves	1 Coconut
10oz Black pepper	10oz Cassava flour
16oz prawns	14oz Mixed seafood
16oz Olive oil	12oz Bacon
10oz Mushrooms	10oz Lime
8oz Thyme	8oz Cilantro
8oz Chili	16oz Beef
14oz Cauliflower	8oz Brussels sprouts
10oz Coconut flour	12oz Kale
8oz psyllium husk powder	8oz Oregano
6oz herbs	12oz Chocolate stick
4 avocados	10oz Peanut butter
14oz olive oil	3 cups Strawberries
12oz baby spinach	3 Pears
16oz smoked salmon	1 cup White wine
16oz turkey breast	16oz crab meat
6 cups Water	8oz coconut milk
10oz rosemary	10oz carrot
8oz garlic powder	8oz bone broth
8oz Sage	6oz multigrain waffles
8oz Chives	6oz maple syrup
12oz Lemon juice	6oz coconut sugar
	6oz chili seasoning mix

6oz Nutritional yeast 8oz Basil 6oz Pine nuts 8oz Coconut flour 6oz Stevia 10oz Baking powder ½ liter Milk 8oz Vanilla extract 14oz Butter	12oz cod filets

Day 22-28

10 Bananas	16oz Spinach
24 oz Lemon juice	10oz Oregano
20oz Raspberry yogurt	Brewed coffee
10ozRaisins	20oz Almond butter
12oz Sunflower kernels	15oz Cacao butter
10oz White fish	24oz Coconut oil
12oz Cilantro	10oz Stevia
14oz Green onions	17oz Vanilla bean
12oz Turmeric	Ice cubes
14oz Garlic cloves	20oz Coconut whipped
14oz Coconut aminos	cream
10oz Coconut milk	12oz Cacao nibs
16oz Salt	8 Avocados
14oz Cinnamon	12 oz Mozzarella
12oz Ginger	12oz Italian seasoning
12oz Ground oil	10oz Balsamic vinegar
10oz Lime juice	20oz Basil
8oz Onion powder	24oz Pork
8oz Garlic powder	10 Lemons
14oz Mushrooms	32oz coconut flour
8oz Paprika	10oz bone broth
14oz Pepper	8oz chives
24oz Beef	8oz brewed decaf
16oz Cheese	10oz hemp hearts
12 Eggs	10oz collagen
8oz Tabasco	16oz broccoli

10oz Mayonnaise	1 grain bread
16oz Smoked salmon	2 duck breasts
12oz Crab claw meat	chicken broth
10oz Green onion	4 oranges
8oz Duck fat	12oz arrowroot flour
14oz Green plantain	20oz ghee
4 Chickens	12oz octane oil
10oz Rice vinegar	14oz romaine lettuce
12oz Black pepper	28oz bacon
8oz Dijon mustard	1 beef roast
10oz Celery	14oz white button mushrooms
12oz Scallions	
18oz Cherry tomatoes	8oz turmeric
12oz Bell peppers	12oz carrots
24oz Flank steak	10oz Strawberries
12oz Fresh parsley	12oz orange juice
20oz Olive oil	16oz lime sauce
20ozAvocado oil	pork carnitas
12oz sour cream	10oz lime juice
14oz fresh dill	16oz plain yogurt

Day 1
Breakfast: *Frittata with Spinach and Mushrooms*

Tasty, simple, and packed with nutrition, this breakfast is best for sharing with a group of people to get your day started.

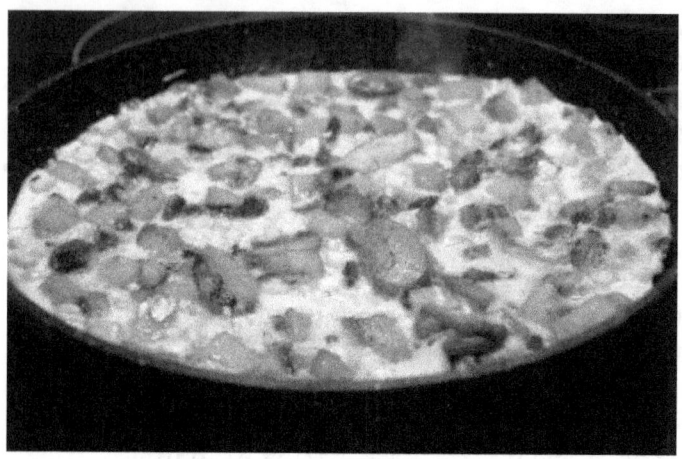

Servings: 6

Ingredients:

- 2 tablespoons Butter
- 6 ounces Bacon, coarsely diced
- 8 ounces Spinach
- 6 Eggs
- 1 cup Heavy Cream
- 6 ounces Shredded Cheese
- Salt & Pepper (to taste)

Directions:

1. Preheat the oven to 350 degrees.
2. Heat 2 tablespoons of butter over medium heat in a frying pan on the stovetop.

3. When heated, add bacon to pan and cook until desired crispiness. Then add the spinach and stir together until soft. Remove both from pan and drain the fat. Set to the side for now.
4. In a separate medium-sized bowl, combine the eggs and cream. Once whisked together, grease a 9x9 baking dish and pour the mixture in.
5. Stir in bacon, spinach, and any shredded cheese. Put dish and mixture in the oven.
6. Bake 30 minutes until perfectly browned.

Per serving: Calories: 561/ Carbs: 4.1 g/ Fat: 59 g/ Protein: 27 g

---

Lunch: *Thai Chicken Noodle Salad*

A delicious chicken noodle salad with fresh herbs changes the taste of your fasting and make it more delicious.

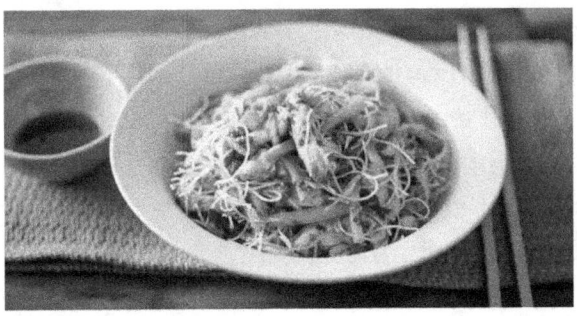

Servings: 4

Ingredients:

For Chicken

- 3 boneless chicken breasts (skinless) cut into strips
- 2 roughly chopped garlic cloves

- 1 big piece fresh ginger, peeled and chopped
- 1 tbsp tamarind
- 2 tbsp soy sauce
- 2 tbsp basil leaves, picked
- 1 lime juice

For Dressing

- 1 tbsp palm sugar
- 1 lime juice
- 2 garlic cloves, crushed
- 1 tbsp dark soy sauce
- 1 tbsp finely grated ginger
- 2 tbsp fish sauce
- 2 finely chopped red chilies

For Salad

- 250g rice noodles
- 1 peeled and julienned carrots
- 2 finely sliced onions
- 2 tbsp basil leaves chopped
- 2 tbsp chopped coriander leaves
- 4 tbsp roasted peanuts
- 2 tbsp chopped mint leaves

Directions:

1. Take a bowl and combine the chicken with marinate ingredients. Cover the mix with cling film and store in a fridge for couple of hours.
2. Place a medium steamer over a large pan of water. Place chicken pieces into the steamer. Cover and steam over 5-6 minutes.

3. Remove chicken from the steamer and repeat the remaining pieces.
4. For dressing, place all ingredients and blend until well combined.
5. For salad, pour boiling water over noodles and soak for 4-5 minutes. Infuse it about 5-10 minutes.
6. Add salad and ingredients. Mix up well.
7. Add chicken to the salad and toss. Finish it with drizzle of remaining dressing.

Per serving: Calories: 312/ Fat: 9 g/ Carbs: 24g/ Protein: 16.8 g

---

Dinner: *Salmon & Veggies*

Seafood is the main source of omega-3. Salmon is one of them and it's a tasty and yummy fish that can also be healthy as a food.

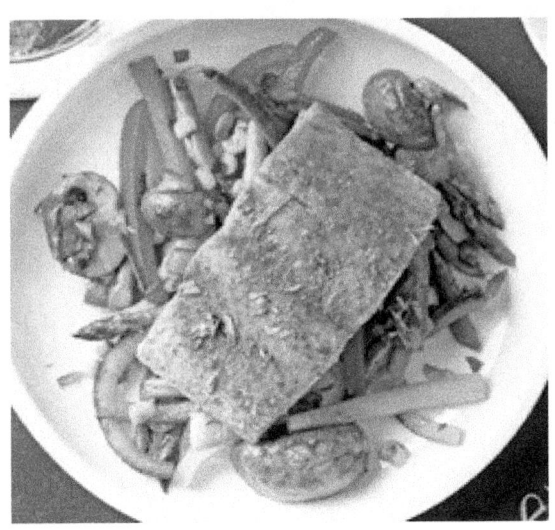

Servings: 3

Ingredients:

- 1-pound salmon
- 2 tbsp ghee
- 2 tbsp fresh lemon juice
- 4 cloves finely diced garlic

Directions:

1. Preheat the oven to 400°F.
2. Mix lemon juice, ghee, and garlic together.
3. Place the Salmon in foil and pour with lemon and ghee mixture over the top.
4. Wrap salmon with the foil paper and place it on a baking sheet.
5. Bake about 15 minutes or until salmon is cooked through.
6. If your oven size allows, then you can roast your vegetables alongside and salmon on a separate baking sheet.

Per serving: Calories: 324/ Carbs: 63 g/ Fat: 11 g/ Protein: 37 g

Day 2
Breakfast: *Pancakes with Berries*

These pancakes have a unique flavor, but they're nutritionally amazing and great for starting your day. This recipe few minutes to prep and cook.

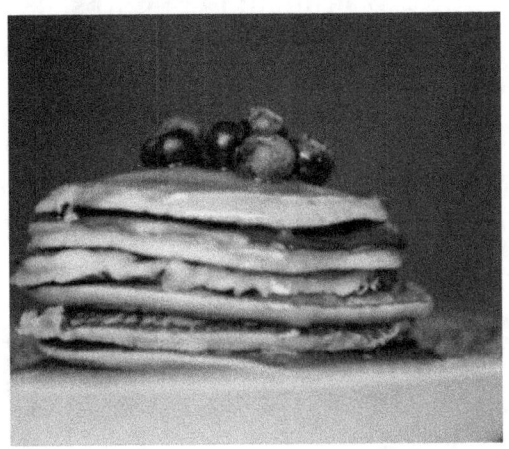

Servings: 4

Ingredients:

- 4 Eggs
- 7 ounces Cheese
- 1 tablespoon Psyllium Husk Powder
- 2 ounces Coconut Oil
- ½ cup Berries, for topping

Directions:

1. In a medium-sized mixing bowl, stir together the first three ingredients and let sit. After about 10 minutes, the mixture should be perfectly thickened.
2. Grab a large-sized non-stick skillet and heat butter or coconut oil until melted. Portion out 0.5-cup scoops of

the batter onto the skillet and cook 4 minutes on each side until done.

3. Prepare berries as desired (sliced or whole, etc.), and top finished pancakes with them for a delightful boost of sweetness.

Per serving: Fat: 39 g/ Protein: 13 g/ Carbs: 5 g/ Calories: 425

Lunch: *Chicken Breast*

There is nothing easier than throwing a nice chicken breast together. The chicken will provide you with enough protein to keep you full on your fasting days.

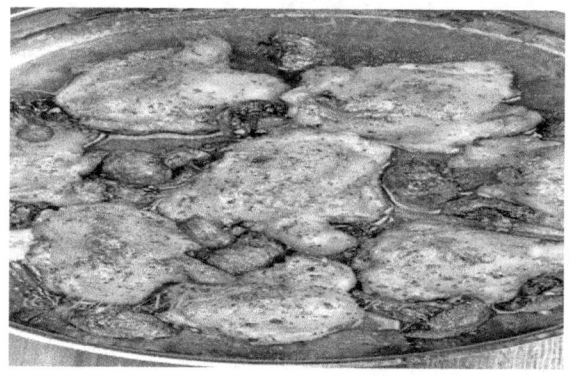

Servings: 2

Ingredients:

Cooking spray

- 2 pieces Chicken breasts
- Salt
- Pepper
- ½ tsp Italian seasoning
- 1 tbsp Balsamic vinegar

- 2 Tbsp cheese
- 1 Sliced tomato

Directions:

1. Turn on the oven to a broil setting. Take out your broiler pan and spray it with some cooking spray.
2. Rinse the chicken off and then blot dry with some paper towels. Season the chicken with the pepper, salt, and Italian seasoning.
3. Lay the chicken onto your prepared broiler pan and then broil for 5 minutes on each side until the chicken reaches 165 degrees.
4. Place two tomato slices on each chicken breast and add the cheese to the top. Spoon the balsamic vinegar over it all.
5. Place this back into the oven and let it broil for another 3 minutes until the cheese is a pale brown. Plate dish and serve.

Per serving: Calories: 220/ Carbs: 11 g/ Fat: 12 g/ Protein: 23 g

---

Dinner: *Bacon and Mushrooms with Greens*

With a modest side-salad, this entrée is both elegant and appropriately filling. You'll want to bring it out when friends come around—or even for date night!

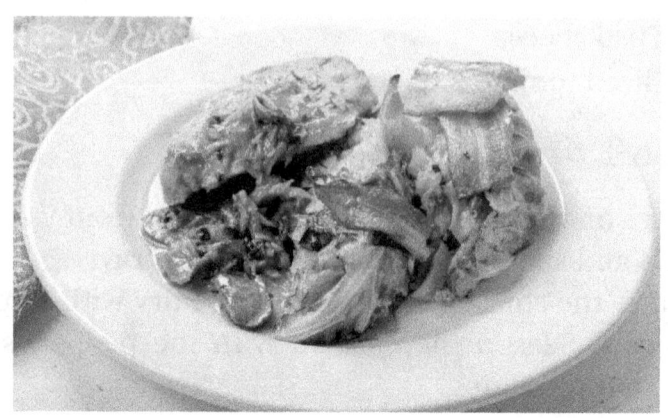

<u>**Servings:** 2</u>

<u>**Ingredients:**</u>

- 4 slices Bacon, cut into half-inch pieces
- 2 cups Mushrooms, halved
- ½ teaspoon Salt
- 2 sprigs fresh herb Thyme, destemmed
- 3 Garlic cloves, minced
- 2 cups Greens of your choice
- ¼ cup Salad Dressing

<u>**Directions:**</u>

1. Assemble the side-salad quickly by taking your choice of greens and sprinkling on a bit of dressing. Set aside or place in the refrigerator for just a few moments.
2. Take a large-sized skillet and bring to medium heat. Add bacon and cook until desired crispiness is reached. Stir in mushrooms and bring to browned color.
3. Stir in salt, thyme leaves, and garlic. Cook 5 minutes then serve hot alongside your salad.

Per serving: Calories: 257/ Carbs: 8.4 g/ Fat: 14 g/ Protein: 15 g

Day 3
Breakfast: *Home-Made Granola Bars*

This is a great bar to make upfront and then store them in an airtight container – don't overload yourself on them.

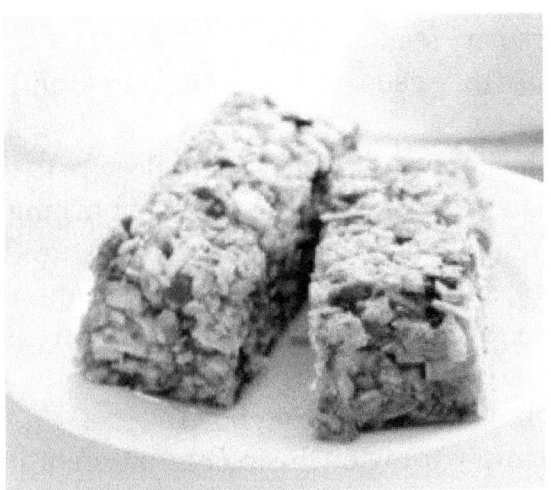

Servings: 5

Ingredients:

- ½ cup raw almonds, roughly chopped
- 2 tablespoons chia seeds
- 2 tablespoons flax seeds
- 2 tablespoons sunflower seeds
- ¼-cup organic peanut butter
- 2 tablespoons hemp seeds
- 1½ cups oats
- 1 cup of dates
- ¼ cup honey

Directions:

1. Preheat the oven to about 180-degrees Celsius.
2. Toast both the almonds, along with the oats, for a maximum of 15 minutes.
3. Put the dates up into a food processor and process until they are very small pieces.
4. Now mix the seeds, the oats, the dates, and the almonds in one bowl.
5. Place the honey into a saucepan. Be sure to turn the stove top up to a low heat setting to avoid burning the mixture.
6. Add the peanut butter. Once the mixture is warm and starts to combine, stir it once or twice and then pour the mixture over the seeds and oats mixture that you previously combined. Thoroughly mix the combination that is now in your mixing bowl.
7. Now, simply transfer this combination of ingredients to an appropriate dish, cover the dish with some plastic wrap. Be sure to squeeze down on the mixture that is now in the dish in order to compress them.
8. Allow the mixture to cool in the freezer for about 20 minutes. Remove and then cut it up into 10 bars of equal size.

Per serving: Calories: 238/ Fat: 9 g/ Carbs: 9 g/ Protein: 6.8 g

---

Lunch: *Pork Carnitas*

These pork carnitas are quick and easy to make. You can always save yourself time by making extra pork and freezing it - you'll thank yourself later when you feel tired from a busy day and the only thing you'll have to do is reheat your leftovers.

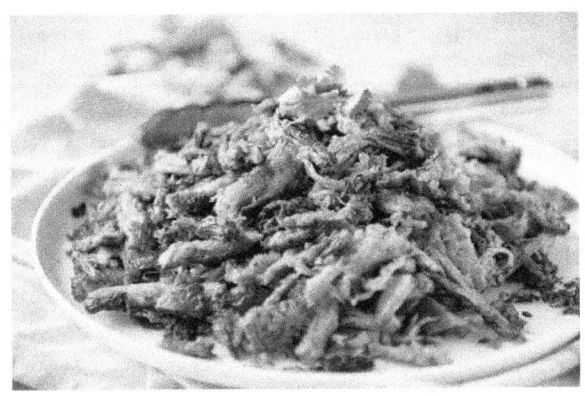

Servings: 4

Ingredients:

- 0.5 lb. Pork tenderloin
- Pepper
- ¼ tsp Salt
- ½ tbsp Dark molasses
- ½ tbsp Orange juice
- 1 Tbsp sugar
- 1 Minced garlic clove

Directions:

1. Rinse off the pork tenderloin and blot it down with some paper towels. Slice thinly and then set it aside.
2. Place a skillet on a flame or burner set to high, and then heat it up for about a minute. Once the skillet is hot, add the pork tenderloin. Cook these for about 4 minutes until the pork is tender and cooked throughout.
3. Drain out the oil before stirring in the pepper, salt, molasses, orange juice, and sugar.
4. Stir this around and simmer until your sauce is thick. Turn off the heat and let it stand for a few minutes to thicken before serving.

Dinner: *Curry Chicken Lettuce-Wraps*

With a little effort, these lettuce-wraps are just as delicious than you can imagine! There is a little less fat in this recipe and you can't fail to like it!

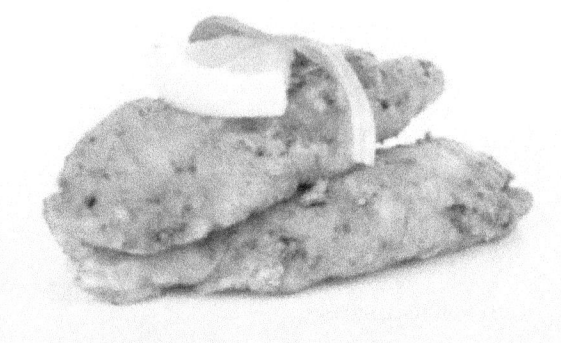

Servings: 2

Ingredients:

- 1 pound, boneless & skinless Chicken Breasts
- ¼ cup Onion, minced
- 2 cloves Garlic, minced
- 2 teaspoons Curry Powder
- 1½ teaspoons Salt
- 3 tablespoons Butter
- 1 cup Cauliflower Rice
- Lettuce leaves, cut into halves
- ¼ cup Sour Cream

Directions:

1. Start by preparing your chicken thighs; cut them into one-inch pieces.
2. Take a large-sized skillet and heat 2 of the 3 tablespoons of butter on the skillet at medium heat. Add onion and cook till soft and browned.
3. Stir in chicken pieces, garlic, and salt. Cook for about 10 minutes.
4. Stir in the last tablespoon of butter, curry powder, and cauliflower rice. Cook about 5 minutes longer.
5. Serve in lettuce leaves or half-wraps, and top with a scoop of cream! Enjoy.

Per serving: Calories: 554/ Carbs: 7.2 g / Fat: 36.4 g/ Protein: 50.9 g

Day 4
Breakfast: *Quiches Breakfast*

Quiches are easy to make, and they are perfect if you're on the go. Perfect for breakfast or a mid-day snack, these quiches have all the protein you need to stay satisfied all day long.

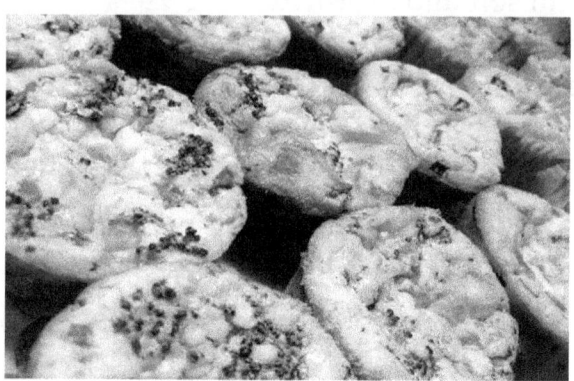

Servings: 5

Ingredients:

- 2 tsp Olive oil
- ¼ tsp Pepper
- ½ tsp Salt
- 1 Tbsp Rosemary
- ¾ cup Parmesan cheese
- 5 Egg whites
- 5 Eggs
- Cooking spray
- 3 oz. Baby spinach
- 6 oz Mushrooms
- 1 Minced garlic clove
- 1 Chopped onion

Directions:

1. Turn on the oven and allow it to heat up to 350 degrees. Coat some muffin tins with cooking spray and add some liners into each one.
2. In a bowl, whisk together the pepper, salt, rosemary, Parmesan cheese, egg whites, and eggs to make them fluffy.
3. Take out a skillet and heat up the olive oil inside. Add the garlic and onion and cook a couple minutes to release their aroma. Now, add the mushrooms and cook for another 5 minutes.
4. Take the pan off the heat and let it cool down a little bit. Place some of this mixture into each of the prepared muffin cups and add some spinach on the top.
5. Slowly pour the egg mixture into each cup and fill to the rim. Add these to the oven and let them bake.
6. After 25 minutes, take them out of the oven and allow them to cool down before serving.

Per serving: Calories: 83/ Carbs: 2 g/ Fat: 5 g/ Protein: 8 g

---

Lunch: *Pulled Pork Sliders*

With its homemade sauce and perfect tenderness, this slider will make you feel gleeful and packed with energy to keep your intermittent fast going strong for the rest of the day.

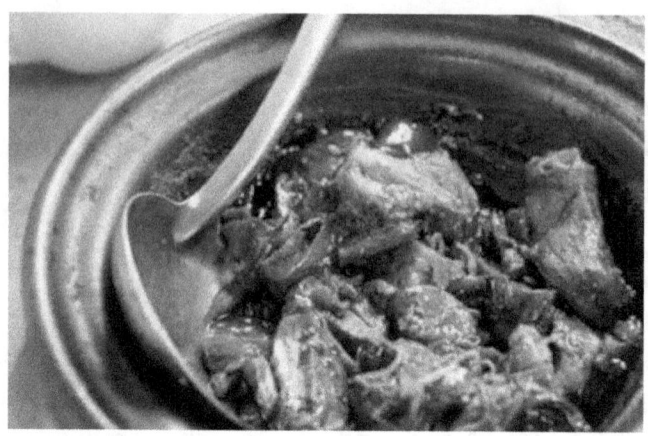

Servings: 4

Ingredients:

- 3 pounds Pork Roast, boneless, cut into inch pieces
- 1 tablespoon Butter
- 2 teaspoons Salt
- 2 teaspoons Garlic Powder
- 1 teaspoon Onion Powder
- 1 teaspoon Black Pepper
- 1 tablespoon Smoked Paprika
- 2 tablespoons Tomato Paste
- ½ cup Apple Cider Vinegar
- 2 tablespoons Coconut Aminos
- ½ cup Bone Broth
- ¼ cup Butter, melted

Directions:

1. Trim any fat from your pork roast and then cut it into appropriate chunks.

2. In a small-sized bowl, combine salt, paprika, pepper, onion and garlic powders and then rub the mixture onto the pork.
3. Grab a large-sized skillet and melt the tablespoon of butter before adding your chunks of pork to the skillet as well.
4. In a separate, medium-sized bowl, combine all other ingredients and pour over the pork in the skillet.
5. Boil the mixture to start then simmer for 30 minutes until meat is tender and is easy to pull apart in the sauce.
6. Serve on low-carb bread alternative or eat in portions alone.

Per serving: Calories: 184/ Fat: 15.1 g/ Carbs: 3.6 g/ Protein: 9.1 g

---

Dinner: *Single-Pan Fajita Steak*

With just one sheet pan, this recipe comes together quickly and packs quite the punch for flavor! This dish is sure to please.

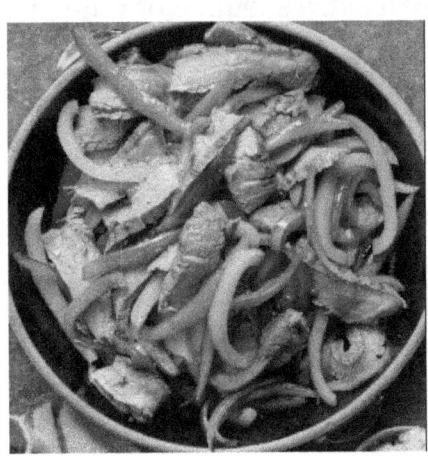

Servings: 5

Ingredients:

- 2 cloves Garlic minced
- 1 medium Onion, sliced thinly
- ½ tsp Chili Powder
- 1 tablespoon Cumin
- Salt and Pepper
- ¼ cup Coconut Oil
- 1 Lime, juiced & zested
- 1 Lemon, juiced & zested
- 1 sliced Yellow Pepper
- 1-pound Beef Steak, sliced into strips
- 1 thinly sliced Red Pepper

Directions:

1. Prepare the meat and vegetables and then stir all ingredients together on a lined or greased baking sheet.
2. Preheat oven to 350 degrees then bake for 15 minutes. Half-way through the process, stir the mixture well.
3. Serve with an extra sprinkle of lime juice.

Per serving: Calories: 440/ Carbs: 5 g/ Fat: 33 g/ Protein: 31 g

Day 5
Breakfast: *Spinach Frittata*

This recipe is easy to prepare and it doesn't have many ingredients. It is very nutritious and it gives you energy throughout the day.

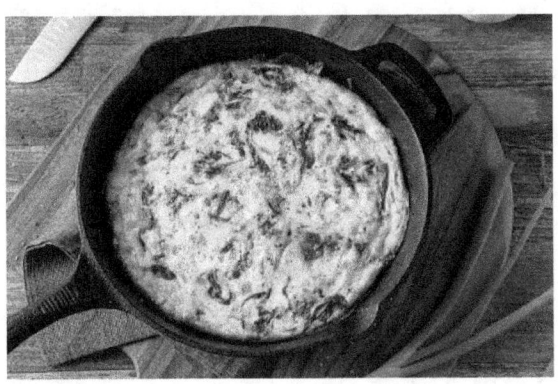

Servings: 4

Ingredients:

- 5oz bacon, diced into small pieces
- 2 tbsp butter
- 8oz spinach, fresh if possible
- 8 eggs
- 5oz cheese, shredded
- 1 cup of heavy whipping cream
- Salt
- Pepper
- Greased baking dish (oven proof)

Directions:

1. Preheat your oven to 175°C.
2. Melt the butter in the pan and cook the bacon until it is as crispy as you like.

3. Transfer the spinach to the pan and stir well until it has wilted slightly. Place the pan to one side and turn off the heat.
4. Into a separate bowl, combine the eggs and cream. Pour the egg mixture into a baking dish (pre-greased).
5. Top the mixture with the cheese, spinach, and bacon.
6. Place the dish into the oven and cook for 25 minutes.
7. Serve and enjoy!

Per serving: Calories: 513/ Carbs: 6.3 g/ Fat: 54 g/ Protein: 31 g

---

Lunch: *Easy Chicken Salad*

With a bread substitute of your choosing or over greens, this chicken salad will do just the trick. It even adds an interesting flavor spin on the traditional chicken salad that you can either appreciate or alter to your preferences.

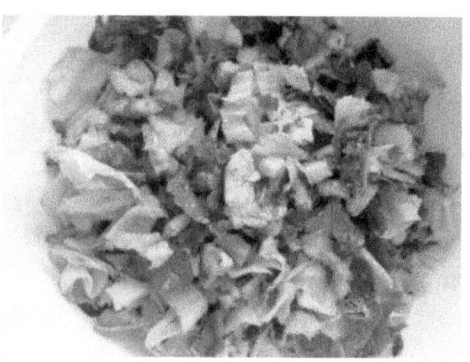

Servings: 6

Ingredients:

- 1.5-pound Chicken Breast
- 3 Celery stalks, sliced
- ½ cup Mayo

- 2 teaspoons Brown Mustard
- ½ teaspoon Salt
- 2 tablespoons fresh Dill, chopped
- ¼ cup Pecans, chopped

Directions:

1. Heat the oven to 425 degrees and line a baking sheet with parchment paper, aluminum foil, or baking spray.
2. Add chicken breast and cook until done throughout. This will take about 15 minutes.
3. Cool the breast completely. This can take anywhere from 10-30 minutes. Once cooled, cut into bite-size pieces.
4. Take a large-sized bowl and stir everything except the dill and pecans together.
5. Cover and chill about 1 hour before adding in dill and pecans. Serve cold.

Per serving: Calories: 279/ Carbs: 1.1 g/ Fat: 19 g/ Protein: 24.8 g

---

Dinner: *Salmon and Light Cream Sauce*

With just a handful of ingredients and a few simple steps, this recipe is gloriously easy and even more delicious than you could ever imagine. Trust me.

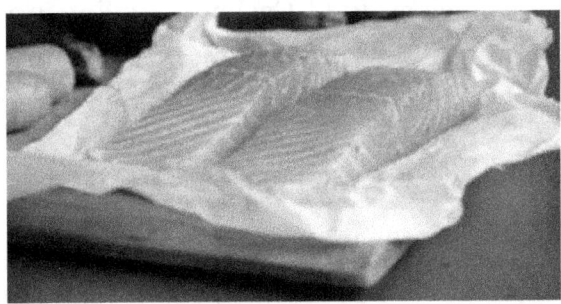

Servings: 6

Ingredients:

- 2 tablespoons Olive Oil
- 3 6-ounce fillets Salmon Fillets
- 2 cloves Garlic, minced
- 1-ounce Cream Cheese
- 2 tablespoons Capers
- 1 tablespoon Lemon Juice
- 2 teaspoons fresh Dill
- 2 tablespoons Parmesan Cheese, grated

Directions:

1. Grab a medium-sized skillet and heat the oil to start. Add the salmon fillets once heated through and cook 5 minutes on each side.
2. Set fish aside to get the sauce together.
3. In that same pan, add garlic and cook on medium heat for 2 minutes. Add cream cheese, lemon juice, and capers. Simmer for 5 minutes or until thickened.
4. Once thickening begins, return salmon to pan and spoon the sauce over each of the fillets.
5. On low heat now, bring the salmon to the appropriate temperature. Garnish with dill and parmesan and serve!

Per serving: Calories: 494/ Carbs: 2 g/ Fat: 30 g/ Protein: 54 g

Day 6
Breakfast: *Green Smoothie*

You will want to go for this green smoothie instead of take a high-sugar fruit smoothie to avoid the starting your day on a blood-sugar roller coaster.

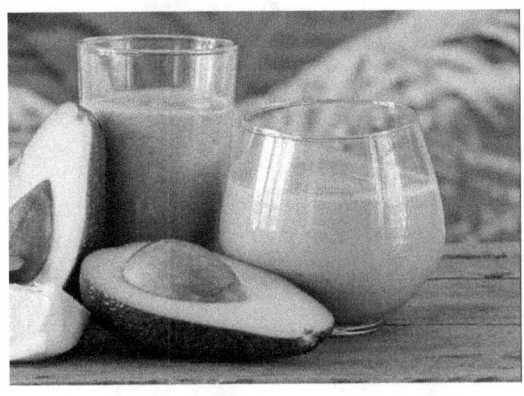

Servings: 2

Ingredients:

- 1 avocado
- 1 small handful blueberries
- 1 cup coconut milk
- 1 tablespoon chia seeds
- 1 cup kale

Directions:

1. Blend all ingredients in a blender until smooth.

Per serving: Calories: 459/ Carbs: 11.4 g/ Fat: 33 g/ Protein: 66 g

Lunch: *Pesto Turkey Meatballs*

This is full of flavor and it is an easy-to-make recipe. It is made with only 5 ingredients which makes it relatively easy. The meatballs are so versatile and delicious.

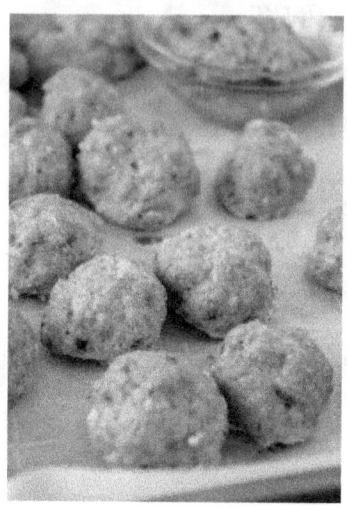

Servings: 8

Ingredients:

- 32 oz ground turkey
- ½ cup fresh basil
- ¼ cup olive oil
- ¼ cup fresh chives
- 1 lemon, zest and juice

Directions:

1. Preheat oven to 375°F. Use aluminum foil to line a rimmed baking sheet.
2. Blend together chives, basil, olive oil, lemon zest and juice in a blender until smooth.

3. Mix together pesto mixture and turkey in large bowl. Roll into balls and arrange on the baking sheet.
4. Bake for 25-30 minutes and serve while warm.

Per Serving: Calories: 230/ Fat: 15.7 g/ Carbs: 0.5 g/ Protein: 22.4 g

---

Dinner: *Parmesan Bacon-Asparagus Roll-Ups*

With the perfect touches of sweetness from the maple-flavored syrup and char from the baking process, these roll-ups are either the best treat ever or the perfect small meal.

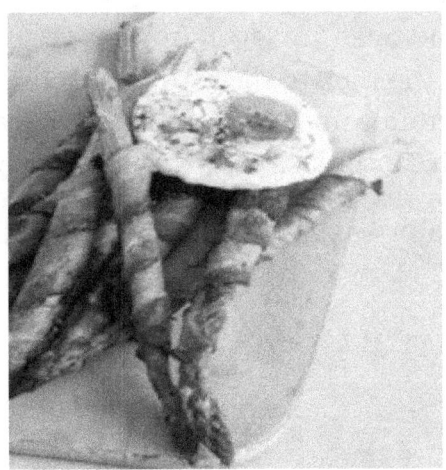

Servings: 2

Ingredients:

- ½ cup Maple-Flavored Syrup
- ½ cup Butter
- ½ tsp Salt
- ¼ tsp Black Pepper
- 2 pounds Asparagus, washed & ends removed
- 8 slices Bacon

Directions:

1. Start by preheating oven to 425 degrees.
2. Then, grab a small-sized pot and bring it to medium-low heat on the stove top. Add syrup, butter, salt, and pepper. Whisk together until smooth and heated through. Set aside for later.
3. Divide your 2 pounds of asparagus into 8 equal-sized groups. Wrap each group with a strip of bacon and secure the ends with toothpicks, as needed.
4. Line greased baking sheet with asparagus/bacon bundles then pour over with syrup mixture and half the parmesan.
5. Bake in the oven for 30 minutes. Then, switch to broil and bring the rack to the top shelf of the oven.
6. Broil 2 minutes until crispy and partially-charred.
7. Serve with toothpicks removed and enjoy!

Per serving: Calories: 257/ Carbs: 2.8 g/ Fat: 23 g/ Protein: 7 g

Day 7
Breakfast: *Scones*

With these scones, you'll have the perfect excuse to satisfy your sweet tooth without feeling guilty. These scones are packed full of nutritious ingredients like Greek yogurt, whole-grains, and blueberries.

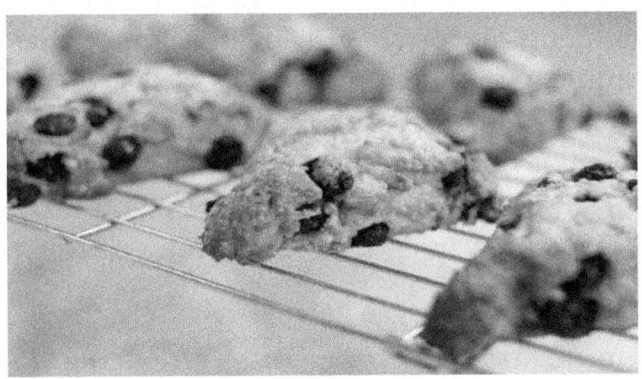

Servings: 3

Ingredients:

- ½ tsp Salt
- 4 tsps. Baking powder
- ¾ cup Whole-wheat flour
- 1¼ cup Flour
- Cooking spray
- 1 cup Wild blueberries
- 1 tsp Vanilla
- ½ cup Milk
- 1 cup Greek yogurt
- 3 Tbsps. Canola oil
- 1 Egg
- ½ cup Sugar
- ¼ cup Baking powder

Directions:

1. Allow the oven to heat up to 400 degrees. Take out two baking sheets and cover with cooking spray.
2. In a bowl, sift together both the flours with the baking soda, salt, and baking powder.
3. In a second bowl, add the vanilla, milk, yogurt, oil, egg, and sugar. Fold the dry ingredients in with the wet ingredients until mixed. Add the blueberries last and continue to mix well.
4. Place a generous spoonful of the batter onto the baking sheets, leaving empty space between each scone. Place the baking pans into the oven for 15 minutes.
5. Remove the scones from the oven and let them cool before serving.

Per serving: Calories: 160/ Carbs: 26 g/ Fat: 4 g/ Protein: 5 g

---

Lunch: *Roasted Beets and Sweet Potatoes*

This recipe is an ideal side dish for everyone in the family. It is easy to prepare as there are few ingredients involved. It can also be used making vegetable wraps.

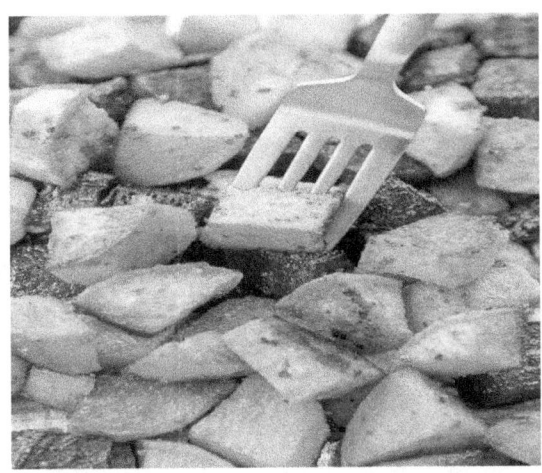

Servings: 5

Ingredients:

- 2 medium beets, peeled and cut into bite size pieces
- ½ teaspoon garlic powder
- ½ teaspoon onion powder
- 5 medium sweet potato, peeled and cut into bite size pieces
- 1 tablespoon coconut oil
- 1 teaspoon sea salt

Directions:

1. Preheat the oven to 400°F.
2. Line a parchment paper on a cookie sheet and place the chopped potatoes and beets. Drizzle oil and add seasonings and mix.
3. Bake in the oven for 20 minutes and toss.
4. Bake for 20 more minutes.
5. Serve and enjoy.

Per serving: Calories: 424/ Carbs: 30.4 g/ Fat: 6 g/ Protein: 16 g

---

<u>Dinner:</u> *Spaghetti Squash*

You're bound to be as amazed as I was when you try this spaghetti squash recipe. Picky eaters will surprise themselves by how much they like it

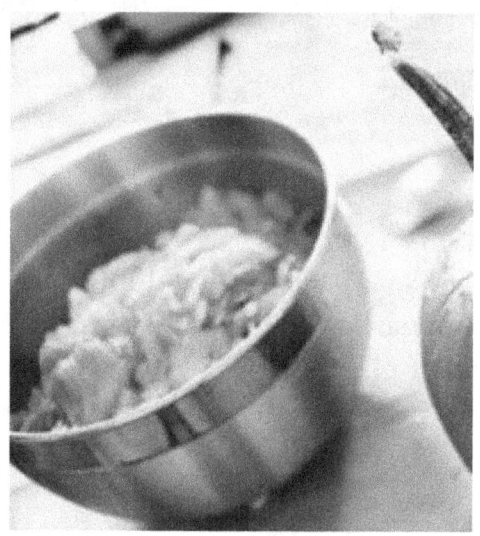

<u>Servings:</u> 4

<u>Ingredients:</u>

- 3 pounds Spaghetti Squash
- 3 cloves Garlic, minced
- 1 teaspoon Olive Oil
- ½-pound Spinach, chopped
- ½ cup Heavy Cream
- ½ cup Parmesan Cheese
- Salt and Pepper

Directions:

1. First, preheat the oven to 400 degrees.
2. Prepare the spaghetti squash by cutting it in half (lengthwise) and pulling out any seeds.
3. Line a baking sheet or grease it and lay spaghetti squash with the cut side down on the sheet. Roast 30-40 minutes until easily stabbed through with a fork.
4. Meanwhile, prepare the sauce. In a medium-sized pot, heat olive oil and garlic for no more than 5 minutes. Stir in spinach, cream, and parmesan in turn.
5. Season with salt and pepper and set aside.
6. When squash has finished roasting, pull it out from oven and begin to pull apart the strands of the squash itself (its name should make sense to you now if it didn't already!).
7. With the squash threads freed, pour the cheese mixture onto the squash and into the inner "boat" part. Top with extra parmesan, as desired, then bake at 350 degrees for 20 additional minutes.
8. At the last second, switch oven to broil and bring cheese to a beautiful browned color. Enjoy hot!

Per serving: Calories: 274/ Carbs: 3.1 g/ Fat: 24.4 g/ Protein: 8 g

Day 8
<u>Breakfast:</u> *Walnut and Apple Loaf*

Made with healthy ingredients, you can enjoy this tasty treat without worrying that you might consume too many calories.

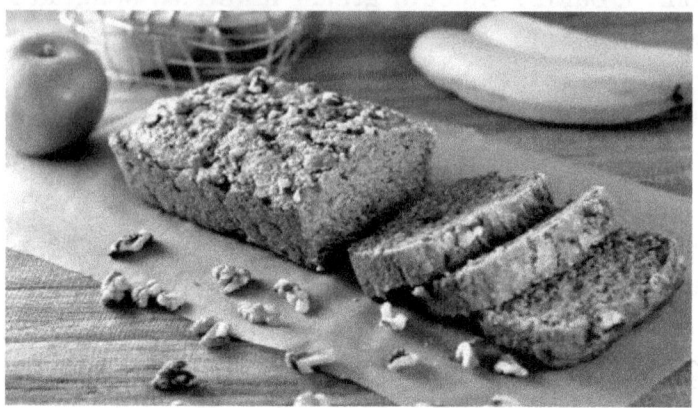

<u>Servings:</u> 4

<u>Ingredients:</u>

- ½ cup Applesauce
- ½ tsp Cinnamon
- ½ tsp Salt
- 1 tsp Baking soda
- 1 cup All-purpose flour
- 1 cup Whole-wheat flour
- Cooking spray
- ½ cup Chopped walnuts
- 1 Chopped apple
- ½ cup Unsweetened almond milk
- 1 Egg
- ½ cup Honey

Directions:

1. Allow the oven to heat up to 325 degrees. Prepare a loaf pan with some cooking spray.
2. Take out a medium bowl and sift together the all-purpose and whole-wheat flours with the cinnamon, salt, and baking soda.
3. In another bowl, combine the honey and applesauce and stir it together until well mixed. Add the almond milk and egg and stir well.
4. Fold the dry ingredients into this but be careful about overmixing. Fold in the walnuts and the apples in as well, making sure to distribute them throughout the batter.
5. Pour this batter into a loaf pan and spread it out evenly. Add this to the oven and allow to bake for almost an hour.
6. After 55 minutes, remove the pan from the oven and let cool for at least 5 minutes before cutting into slices.

Per serving: Calories: 206/ Carbs: 45 g/ Fat: 2 g/ Protein: 5 g

---

Lunch: *Bacon and Green Onion Mashed Cauliflower*

This recipe is packed with ingredients which are a great source of flavor, nutrients and vitamins! It is an ideal meal to carry along to an upcoming party.

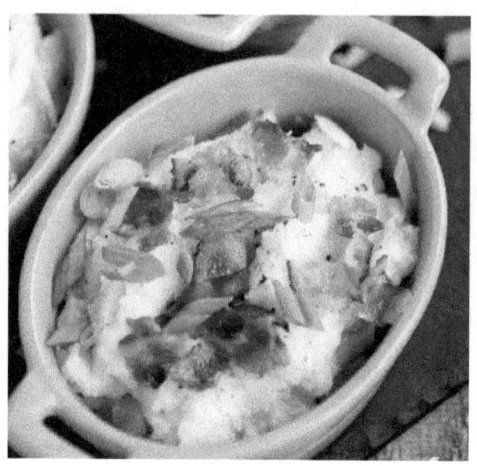

Servings: 4

Ingredients:

- 5 slices of bacon, cooked & crumbled
- 3 tablespoons ghee
- 2 minced garlic cloves
- 5 cups cauliflower florets
- Salt
- 2 sliced onions
- Freshly ground black pepper

Directions:

1. Bring to boil water filled in a large saucepan.
2. Add cauliflower and allow about 15-20 minutes to simmer and drain the water.
3. Put cauliflower back to the saucepan and add garlic, ghee and season.
4. Use a hand mixer and blend cauliflower until smooth.
5. Serve and top with bacon and green onions.

Per serving: Calories: 307/ Carbs: 9.9 g/ Fat: 20 g/ Protein: 43 g

---

Dinner: *Roasted Sweet Potatoes and Brussels Sprouts*

This recipe is nearly in every way superior. It is ideal for holidays and they can be a common thing for your oven during the holidays.

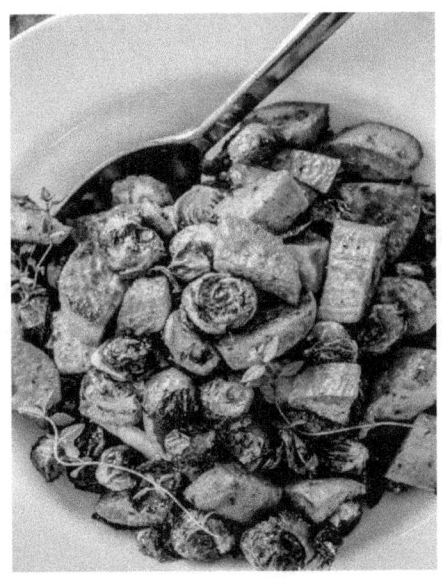

Servings: 6

Ingredients:

- 1 medium sweet potato, peeled and chopped into 1" pieces
- 1-pound Brussels sprouts, trimmed and brown ends cut
- 2 smashed cloves garlic
- 1/3 cup olive oil
- ¼ teaspoon salt

- 1 tablespoon red wine vinegar
- ¼ teaspoon pepper to taste
- Fresh thyme
- 1 teaspoon cumin

Directions:

1. Preheat the oven to 400°F.
2. Add Brussels, sweet potato and garlic into a large bowl and pour the olive over the bowl.
3. Add pepper salt, garlic salt and cumin and stir.
4. Line a foil on a baking sheet pan.
5. Grease the baking sheet pan with some little olive oil.
6. Add the vegetables to the pan and roast for 40-45 minutes, or until brown.
7. Serve in a bowl and use red wine vinegar to toss. Use fresh thyme to garnish and enjoy!

Per serving: Calories: 415/ Carbs: 31.4 g/ Fat: 6 g/ Protein: 40 g

Day 9
Breakfast: *Bananas French Toast*

This is a very nourishing recipe. It is easy to prepare and full of nutrients.

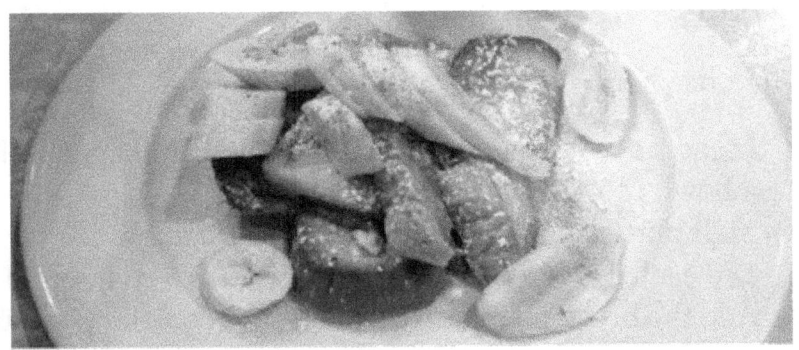

Servings: 4

Ingredients:

The French toast

- 6 slices Challah bread
- 2 eggs
- ½ cup milk
- 1 teaspoon vanilla extract
- ½ teaspoon ground cinnamon
- 3 tablespoons sugar
- Pinch of salt
- Butter, for frying

The Banana Caramel Syrup

- ¼ cup butter
- ¾ cup sugar, lightly packed
- 3 tablespoons whipping (heavy) cream

- ¼ teaspoon ground cinnamon
- 1 teaspoon vanilla extract
- 4 tablespoons dark rum (optional)
- 2 bananas, thickly sliced

Directions:

French toast

1. Mix eggs with sugar, milk, cinnamon, vanilla, and salt in a bowl.
2. Melt butter in a skillet over medium-high heat.
3. Dip each bread slice in the egg mixture to coat well.
4. Add the bread pieces to the skillet and cook for 3 minutes per side until golden brown.
5. Repeat the same steps with the remaining bread slices.
6. Place them on a platter.

Caramel Syrup

1. Heat butter in a pot over medium-high heat.
2. Add brown sugar and whisk well until well combined.
3. Bring the sugar mixture to a boil for 2 minutes.
4. Gradually stir in whipped cream and mix well.
5. Add vanilla and cinnamon. Mix well.
6. Fold in banana slices and rum.
7. Cook for 1 minute.
8. Top the toasted bread slices with this syrup.

Per serving: Calories: 542/ Carbs: 65.3 g/ Fat: 24.2 g/ Protein: 11.1 g

Lunch: *White Beans with Garlic and Basil*

White beans are a great source of nutrition and energy. Try them and you will not be disappointed!

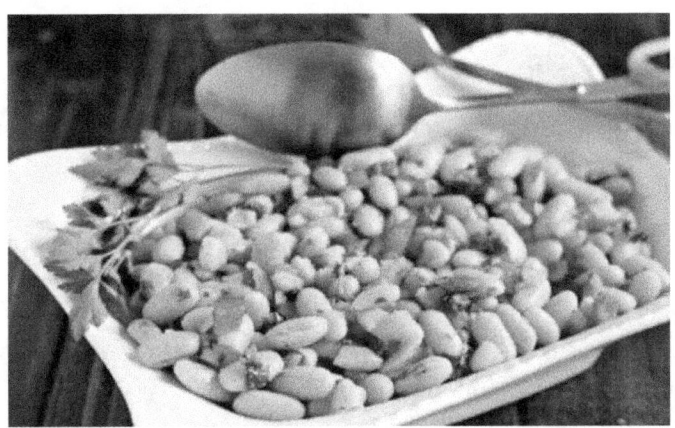

Servings: 2

Ingredients:

- 24 oz. canned rinsed beans
- 1 tablespoon olive oil
- 1½ onion, chopped
- 4 garlic cloves
- 2 quarts vegetable stock
- salt to taste
- 12 oz. (3 medium) fresh tomatoes, peeled and chopped
- 1 large handful of fresh basil
- Juice from 2 lemons
- Freshly ground pepper

Directions:

1. Heat oil in a skillet over medium heat and add garlic and onion.

2. Sauté for 10 to 15 minutes until soft.
3. Drain the rinsed beans and add them to the pan.
4. Stir in tomatoes and cook for 5 minutes.
5. Add the remaining ingredients and stir cook for 5 minutes.
6. Serve warm.

Per serving: Calories: 400/ Carbs: 49.6 g/ Fat: 4.3 g/ Protein: 48.9 g

---

Dinner: *Southern Fried Okra*

This recipe is packed with vegetables which are a great source of flavor, nutrients and vitamins!

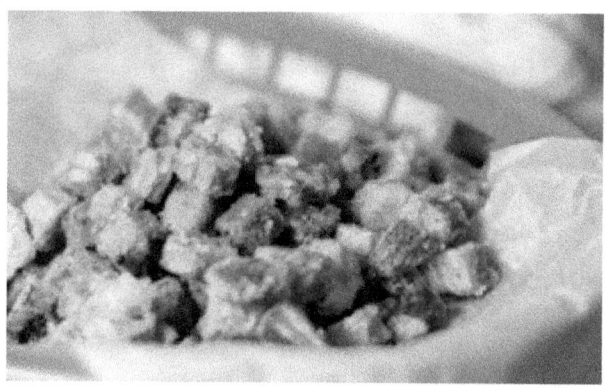

Servings: 3

Ingredients:

- ½ pound fresh okra, stems removed and sliced ¼" thick
- 1 teaspoon onion, granulated
- ¼ cup Cassava Flour
- 3 tablespoons coconut oil
- 2 teaspoons salt
- 2 teaspoons garlic, powder

Directions:

1. Stir seasonings and cassava flour in a bowl to combine. Add in the okra and cover. Shake thoroughly to coat.
2. Heat coconut oil in a pan for 4 minutes. Slowly add okra and cook on each side for about 3-5 minutes, until golden brown.
3. Put the fried okra on a rack lined with paper towels. Allow 5 minutes to cool. Serve and enjoy.

Per serving: Calories: 442/ Carbs: 24.1 g/ Fat: 9 g/ Protein: 24.3 g

Day 10
Breakfast: *Pineapple Pancakes*

Pancakes are a favorite to many. The pineapple gives this recipe a very sweet taste than you just can't turn down!

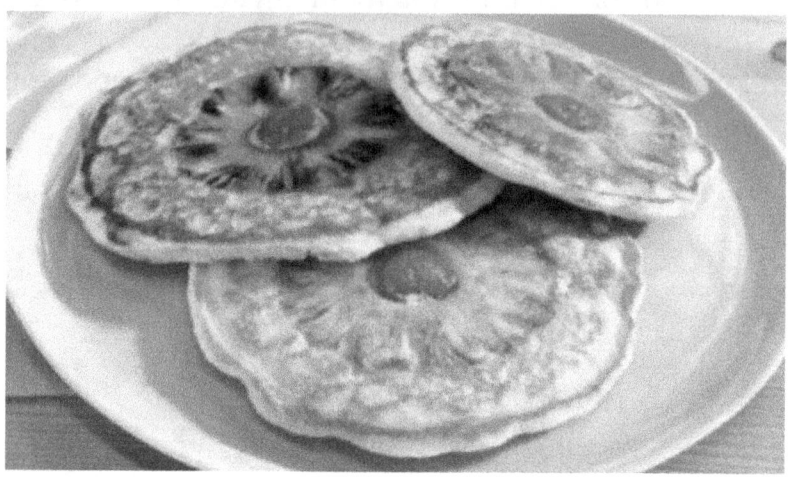

Servings: 3

Ingredients:

- 1⅓ cups all-purpose flour
- 1¼ teaspoons baking powder
- ½ cup packed light brown sugar, separated
- 2 large eggs
- 1 cup buttermilk
- 4 tablespoons melted butter
- 1 teaspoon pure vanilla extract
- ¼ teaspoon ground cinnamon
- Extra butter for your griddle
- 1 (20 ounces) can thinly sliced pineapple
- 8-10 maraschino cherries with stems removed

Directions:

1. Mix flour with baking powder, quarter cup brown sugar in a bowl.
2. Whisk eggs with buttermilk, melted butter, cinnamon, and vanilla extract in another bowl.
3. Add flour mixture to the bowl and mix well until smooth.
4. Heat butter in a nonstick frying pan over medium heat.
5. Place one pineapple ring to the center of the pan.
6. Sprinkle the brown sugar over the pineapple.
7. Cook for 30 seconds until light brown then flip the ring.
8. Place a cherry at the center of the ring.
9. Pour about a quarter cup of flour batter over the pineapple.
10. Cook until firm then flip to cook until golden brown from both the sides.
11. Repeat the process and to use the remaining batter.

Per serving: Calories: 617/ Carbs: 113.9g/ Fat: 13.3 g/ Protein: 14.5 g

---

Lunch: *Cauliflower Fried Rice*

Cauliflower Fried Rice is an amazing recipe filled with lots of flavor that will make you enjoy it. It does not take much time when making it. You will absolutely love this amazing recipe!

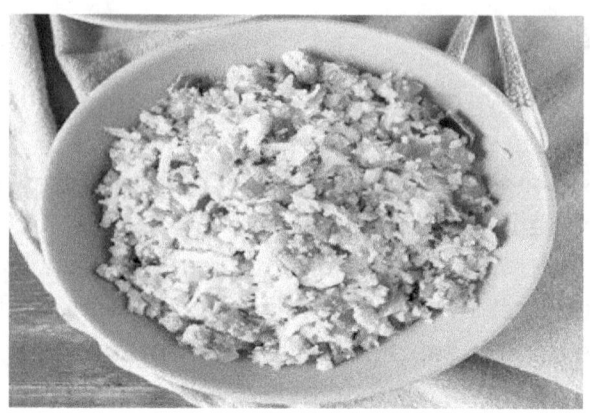

<u>Servings:</u> 6

<u>Ingredients:</u>

- 1 large grated cauliflower
- 1 teaspoon garlic powder
- 2 tablespoons coconut oil
- 1 ½ cup carrots diced
- ½ cup coconut aminos
- 2 large eggs, scrambled
- 1 large diced onion
- 1 teaspoons ginger, ground
- 1 teaspoon salt

<u>Directions:</u>

1. Heat coconut oil in a large pan. Sauté carrots and onions for about 8 minutes until soft.
2. As it cooks, season with garlic, ginger and salt.
3. Add coconut aminos and cauliflower and evenly stir.
4. Cook for 5 more minutes and push the mixture to one side and add the eggs and cook. When cooked, mix.
5. Serve and enjoy!

<u>Per serving:</u> Calories 464/ Carbs 53.2 g/ Fat 9 g/ Protein 12 g

Dinner: *Curly Sweet Potato Fries with Garlic Aioli*

This recipe is crispy and tastes sweet. They are also filled with flavors from the spices that are used in preparation.

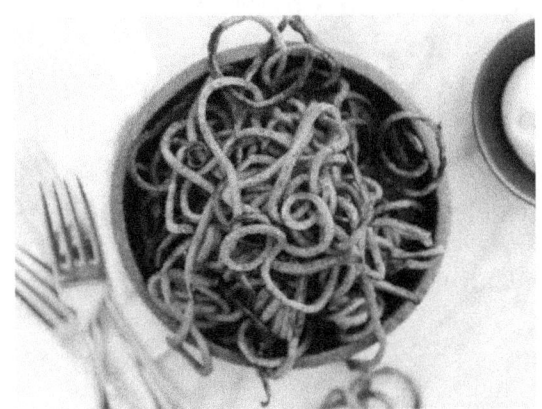

Servings: 2

Ingredients:

Curly Sweet Potato Fries:

- 1 sweet potato
- ½ teaspoon garlic powder
- 1 teaspoon paprika
- 1 tablespoon avocado oil
- Pepper & salt

Garlic Aioli:

- ½ teaspoon lemon juice
- 1 minced garlic clove
- 2 tablespoons mayonnaise
- Pepper & salt

Directions:

1. Preheat the oven to 425°F.
2. Spiralize sweet potato. Put them on a sheet pan and add the spices and oil. Mix together using your hands to coat all sweet potato pieces.
3. Cook in the oven until crispy, or for about 20-25 minutes.
4. Meanwhile, mix to combine all garlic aioli ingredients in a bowl.
5. Serve sweet potato fries with garlic aioli.

Per serving: Calories: 411/ Carbs: 21.3 g/ Fat: 14 g/ Protein: 24 g

Day 11
Breakfast: *Almond and Cherry Cookies*

Who would have thought that cookies can make a healthy breakfast? These small cookies are full of fruit, nuts, and whole grains which provide an excellent source of nutrition in the morning.

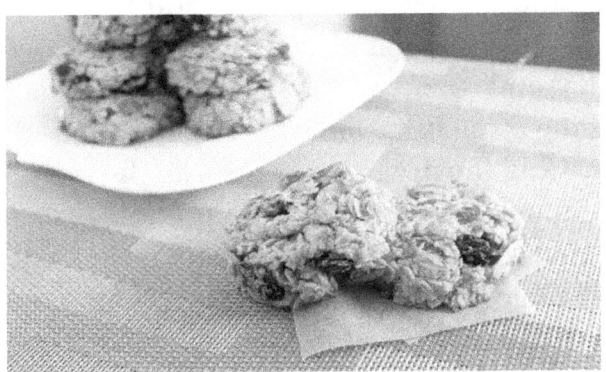

Servings: 6

Ingredients:

- 1 tsp Baking soda
- 2¼ cups Whole-wheat flour
- ½ cup Rolled oats
- Cooking spray
- 1 cup Sliced raw almonds
- 1 cup Chopped tart cherries, dried
- 1 tsp Vanilla
- 2 Eggs
- ½ cup Maple syrup
- ½ cup sugar
- ½ cup Plain Greek yogurt
- ½ cup Applesauce
- ¼ tsp Salt

Directions:

1. Allow the oven to heat up to 350 degrees. Take a few baking sheets and line with some parchment paper.
2. Take out a bowl and combine the salt, baking soda, flour, and oats.
3. In a second bowl, whisk together the Greek yogurt and applesauce. When well mixed, add in the maple syrup and brown sugar and continue to mix well. Add the vanilla and the eggs and mix the ingredients until reaching a smooth even consistency.
4. Slowly fold the dry ingredients into the wet ones and stir to combine. Now, add the almonds and cherries, making sure that they are well distributed in the batter.
5. Add 2 tablespoons of batter onto a baking sheet to make each cookie and then flatten them down a little bit. Place in the oven to bake.
6. After 15 minutes, you can take the cookies out and let them cool before serving or storing.

Per serving: Calories: 214/ Carbs: 36 g/ Fat: 6 g/ Protein: 6 g

---

Lunch: *Spanish Prawns*

This is a delicious recipe that can be taken alongside several main dishes. It is equally easy to prepare as you just put herbs and some rice in pot with broth and it is done!

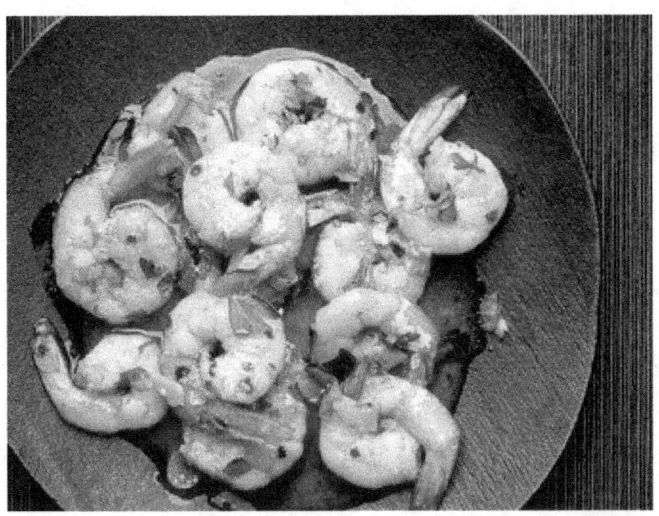

Servings: 2

Ingredients:

- 2 Cloves garlic, peeled and finely chopped
- 1 Fennel bulb thinly sliced
- 1Parsley sprigs
- 5 tablespoons Manzanilla sherry
- 15 Large raw prawns, peeled
- 2 tablespoons Olive oil
- 1 tablespoon Dried tomato paste
- Bread to serve

Directions:

1. Place a large pan over medium heat then add garlic, parsley stalks and fennel then fry for 15 minutes or until tender. Add tomato paste and cherry tomatoes then bring to boil. Cook for 25 minutes until well thickened.
2. Add prawns into the pan then cook for about 2 minutes then turn and cook for another 2 minutes or until pink

all through. Season and sprinkle with parsley leaves then serve with bread.

Per serving: Calories: 171/ Carbs: 8.2 g/ Fat: 15 g/ Protein: 37 g

---

Dinner: *Fried Pickles*

The fried pickles are just amazingly delicious. They are simple and quick to prepare. They are crunchy and filled with nutrients that are good for you.

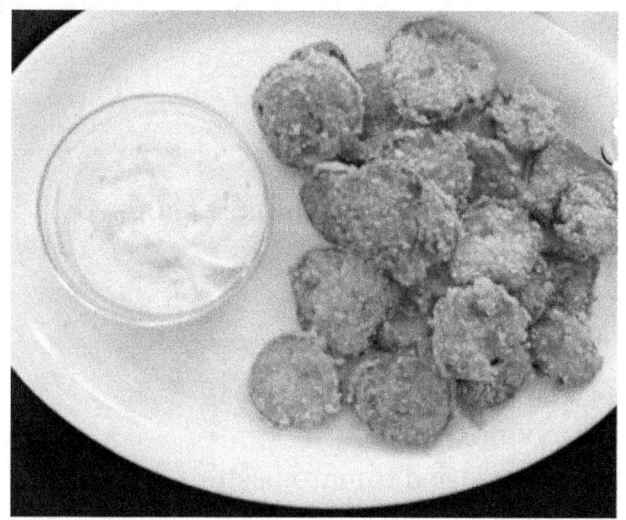

Servings: 4

Ingredients:

- 2½ cups Dill pickles chips
- ¼ teaspoon cayenne pepper
- 6 cups Coconut oil
- Pepper and salt
- ½ cup Almond flour

- ¼ cup Almond Milk
- 1 teaspoon Garlic powder
- 1 large egg
- ½ teaspoon smoked Paprika

Directions:

1. Put coconut oil in a pan and warm it slowly.
2. Meanwhile, drain the pickles and pat them dry with paper towels. Mix the spices and almond flour. Mix egg and almond milk together.
3. When oil starts bubbling, dip several pickles in the egg and almond milk mixture and then into the almond flour mix.
4. Dip into the pan and fry until golden brown or for 2 minutes. Repeat for all remaining pickles.

Per serving: Calories: 293/ Carbs: 12.4 g/ Fat: 8 g/ Protein: 21 g

Day 12
Breakfast: *Chia Pudding*

This amazingly sweet and highly nutritious recipe is easy to prepare and is so ideal for you as breakfast when you start your day

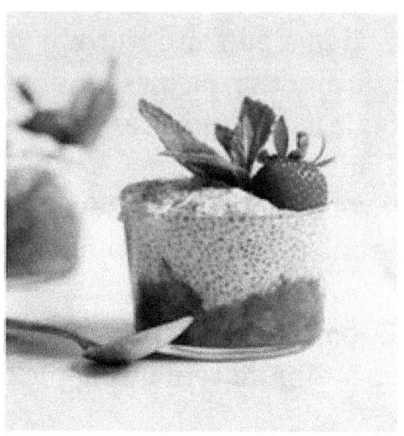

Servings: 1

Ingredients:

- ½ cup dairy-free milk
- 1 tbsp maple syrup
- ½ cup chia seeds
- 1 tsp vanilla extract

Directions:

1. Take a mixing bowl add chia seeds, dairy free milk, maple syrup (to taste), and vanilla extract.
2. Cover it and refrigerate it overnight (or at least 6 hours). The chia pudding should be turned thick and creamy.

Per serving: Calories: 321/ Carbs: 24 g/ Fat: 5 g/ Protein: 18 g

<u>Lunch:</u> *Bang Bang Shrimp*

The Bang Bang Shrimp recipe is flavorful and full of nutrients. It is also easy and quick to prepare. It is creamy, spicy, tender and crispy.

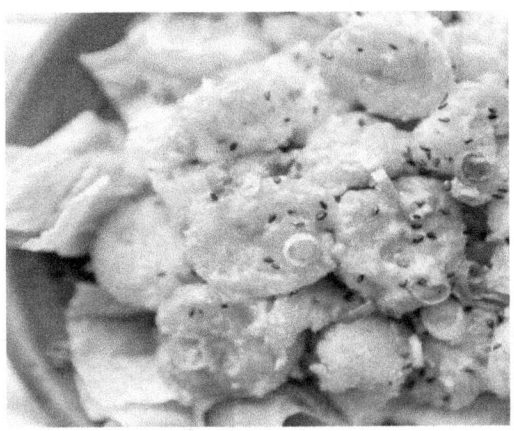

<u>Servings:</u> 4

<u>Ingredients:</u>

Shrimp:

- 1 medium egg, whisk
- ½ cup coconut flour
- coconut oil
- 1-pound shrimp, deveined & peeled
- ½ cup arrowroot powder
- ¼ tsp pepper
- ½ teaspoon salt

Optional:

- Sesame seeds
- 2 sliced onions (green part only)

Bang Bang Sauce:

- 1 minced garlic clove
- 2 teaspoon sriracha
- ¼ cup + 2 tablespoons mayonnaise
- 2 teaspoons coconut aminos
- 2 tablespoon ketchup
- ½ tsp Salt

Directions:

1. Stir all sauce ingredients together and place aside.
2. Whisk arrowroot powder, pepper, salt and coconut flour together in a wide bowl. Add shrimp to eggs and deep in flour and shake off excess. Put on a baking sheet. Do the same for the rest of the shrimp.
3. Heat oil over medium heat in a large skillet. Fry shrimp in batches. Cook until brown and turn the other side. Remove to a plate. Do the same for all shrimp.
4. Toss shrimp in a large bowl with half of sauce. Taste with more sauce. Serve and top with sesame seeds and green onions.

Per serving: Calories: 273/ Carbs: 12.1 g/ Fat: 20 g/ Protein: 43 g

---

Dinner: *Greek-Style Lamb Meatballs*

This recipe is so tasty and you will definitely enjoy it! If you do not love meatballs, it is most likely that you haven't tried these ones yet.

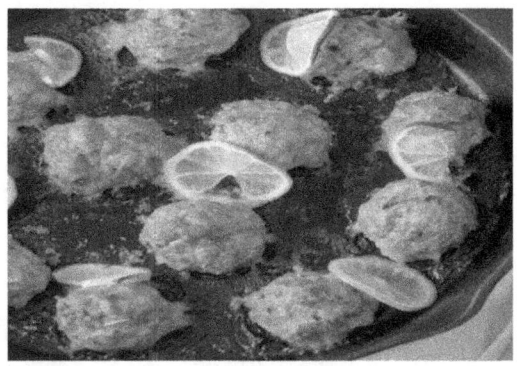

Servings: 3

Ingredients:

- 1-pound ground lamb
- 1 lemon, zested
- 1 tbsp extra virgin olive oil
- ¼ tsp dried oregano
- ¼ tsp black pepper
- ½ tsp sea salt
- ¼ tsp garlic powder
- 1 garlic clove, minced
- ½ fresh lemon, thinly sliced

Directions:

1. Preheat the oven to 400°F.
2. Combine lamb, garlic powder, oregano, black pepper, sea salt, lemon zest and garlic in a mixing bowl.
3. Form meatballs (10-12) using the mixture and put in an oven safe dish. Put lemon slices on the meatballs.
4. Bake in the oven until meatballs are cooked, or for about 20-25 minutes.
5. Sprinkle extra virgin oil on meatballs when served.

Per serving: Calories: 257/ Carbs: 9.2 g/ Fat: 9 g/ Protein: 25g

Day 13
Breakfast: *Fruit Smoothie*

Smoothies are not sweet as milkshake. If you like sweeter then you can add some icing sugar. This smoothie is healthy and tasty too.

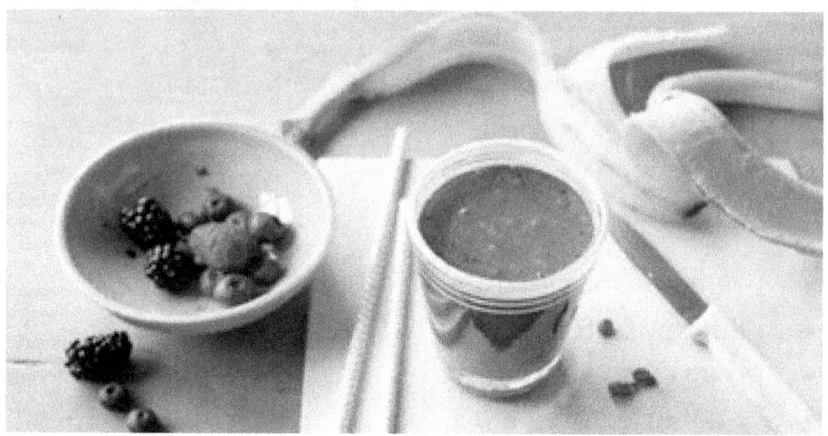

Servings: 2

Ingredients:

- 1 cup fresh blackberries
- 1 ripe medium banana
- 1 cup fresh raspberries
- 1 cup fresh blueberries
- 1 cup milk
- ½ cup pint natural plain yoghurt

Directions:

1. Put all the ingredients into a food processor and process until smooth and serve.

Per serving: Calories: 423/ Carbs: 66 g/ Fat: 4 g/ Protein: 12 g

Lunch: *Fish Salad (Greek Style)*

This recipe is filled with Mediterranean flavors from tomatoes, basil, olives and the simple dressing. It is tasty, fresh and so delicious.

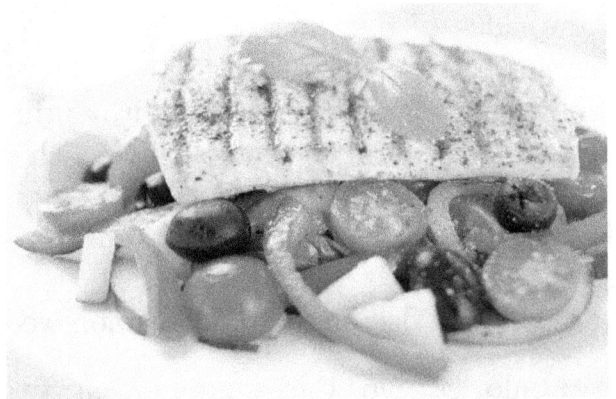

Servings: 2

Ingredients:

- 10 ounces fish
- ½ cup thinly sliced onion
- ½ cup thinly sliced red pepper
- ½ tablespoon oregano, dried
- ½ cup basil
- ½ cup chopped cucumber
- ½ cup cherry tomatoes
- 1 tablespoon olive oil
- ½ cup pitted black olives
- lemon wedge
- pepper and salt

Dressing:

- 1 crushed garlic clove

- 1 tablespoon lemon juice
- 2 tablespoons olive oil
- pepper and salt

Directions:

1. Rub the sides of the fillet with olive oil. Season with pepper and salt and drizzle oregano.
2. Melt olive oil on high heat in a cast iron grill. Once hot, lower heat to medium and cook fish on each side for 3-4 minutes.
3. Add all salad ingredients in a bowl and toss with lemon dressing.
4. Serve salad with fish on top. Add a lemon wedge.

Per serving: Calories: 276/ Carbs: 22.2 g/ Fat: 17 g/ Protein: 54 g

---

Dinner: *Steamed Wild-Caught Crab Legs*

Are you looking for a seafood recipe that is crunchy and can be fixed quickly? Well, look no further. The Steamed Wild-Caught Crab Legs are prepared in just 3 minutes only! It is nourishing and very healthy.

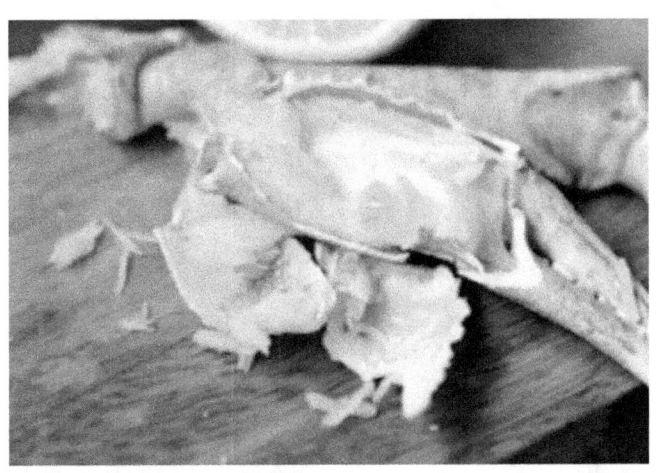

<u>Servings:</u> 4

<u>Ingredients:</u>

- 2 pounds Snow Crab legs, wild-caught
- 1 lemon, sliced
- ¼ cup melted ghee, salted
- 1 cup water

<u>Directions:</u>

1. Put a metal trivet at the base of instant pot and add water.
2. Add crab legs and cover the lid.
3. Press "manual" and set time to 4 minutes.
4. When the instant pot beeps, release pressure and remove the crab legs using tongs.
5. Serve with lemon slices and ghee.

<u>Per serving:</u> Calories: 342/ Carbs: 21.5 g/ Fat: 11 g/ Protein: 42 g

Day 14
Breakfast: *One Pan Breakfast*

This recipe makes a healthy breakfast that will improve metabolism. It will also give you energy to ace the day

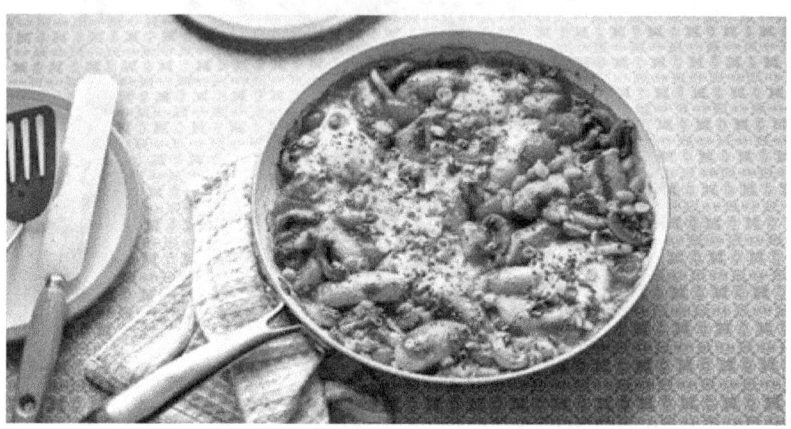

Servings: 3

Ingredients:

- 1 tbsp olive oil
- 4 finely chopped spring onions
- 8 10% fat pork sausages, cut into chunks
- 200g thinly sliced mushrooms
- 4 cherry tomatoes, halved
- ½ garlic cloves, crushed
- 2 large free-range eggs
- ¼ tbsp sweet smoked paprika
- 24oz tin baked beans
- 2 tbsp finely chopped parsley, to garnish

Directions:

1. Take a large frying pan and heat the oil into medium heat. Brown the sausages about 2–3 minutes, then remove from the pan and set aside.
2. Add the mushrooms and spring onions to the pan and cook over a medium heat about 3–4 minutes, or until it softened. Add the garlic and fry about 1 minute. Add the beans, tomatoes and sausages and simmer about 20 minutes or until the sausages are cooked through.
3. Now make four wells in the mixture and crack the eggs into them. Cover the pan and steam about 6–8 minutes, or until the whites get set or cooked to your liking.
4. Scatter a little paprika over each egg, also crumble it over the feta and spoon into the bowls. Garnish it with the parsley and serve.

Per serving: Calories: 353/ Carbs: 22 g/ Fat: 10 g/ Protein: 25 g

---

Lunch: *Oven-baked chicken*

This friendly recipe is made full of flavor and made from ingredients that are free of additives. It also contains all the nutrients that are needed for various body functions.

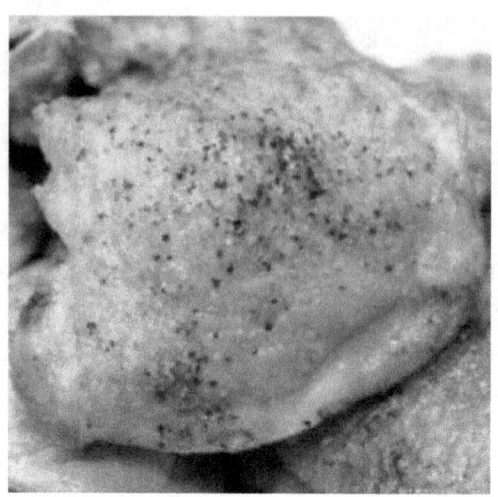

<u>Servings:</u> 4

<u>Ingredients:</u>

- 3 lbs. Whole chicken
- ½ teaspoon Ground black pepper
- 2Minced garlic cloves
- 3 oz Butter
- Salt and pepper

<u>Directions:</u>

1. Get the oven preheated to 4000F then season the chicken with salt and pepper on both the sides.
2. Place the chicken into a baking dish. Place a sauce pan over medium heat then add butter and garlic and cook. Allow the butter to cool for about 3 minutes then pour it inside the chicken.
3. Bake the chicken for one and half hours or until the temperature of the chicken reaches 1800F.
4. Baste the chicken with juices from the bottom of the pan after every 20 minutes.

5. Remove from the oven then serve with juices and preferred side dish.

Per serving: Calories: 753/ Carbs: 1 g/ Fat: 83 g/ Protein: 53 g

---

Dinner: *Rack of Lamb*

This recipe is easy and simple to prepare. It takes little time to have this aromatic recipe ready. To ensure that it comes out perfect, make sure that the lamb is well marinated before you cook.

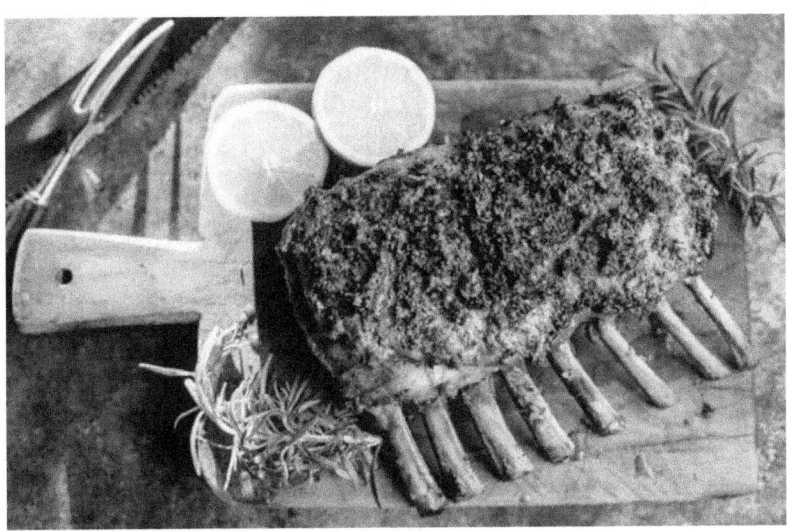

Servings: 4-5

Ingredients:

- 1 frenched rack of lamb (bones exposed)
- Zest from 1 lemon
- 2 teaspoons fresh thyme
- 6 cloves garlic
- ¼ cup olive oil

- 1 tablespoon fresh rosemary
- ¼ cup fresh parsley (optional)
- Pepper and salt

Directions:

1. Preheat the oven to 450°F and set rack in the oven.
2. Use paper towel to pat dry the lamb and put it on a sheet paper.
3. Blend pepper, salt, garlic, parsley, thyme, rosemary and olive oil in a food processor to form a thick pesto. Add lemon zest and zest.
4. Season the lamb with pepper and salt. Rub the mixture on the lamb and let sit for about 50-60 minutes at room temperature.
5. Roast the lamb in the oven for 15 minutes and turn over and roast for about 10-15 minutes.
6. Move the roasted rack to a carving board. Let sit for 10 minutes.
7. Carve the lamb using a knife. Serve an enjoy!

Per serving: Calories: 257/ Carbs: 8.4 g/ Fat: 14 g/ Protein: 15 g

Day 15
Breakfast: *Keto Oatmeal Pancake*

This meal contains rolled oats which are very paramount to the body as it contains a powerful soluble fiber called Beta Glycan which lowers cholesterol levels and improves blood sugar. In addition, it is quite filling and may help you lose weight. Eggs also contain proteins for energy while the cottage cheese adds some more to the healthy nature of the meal.

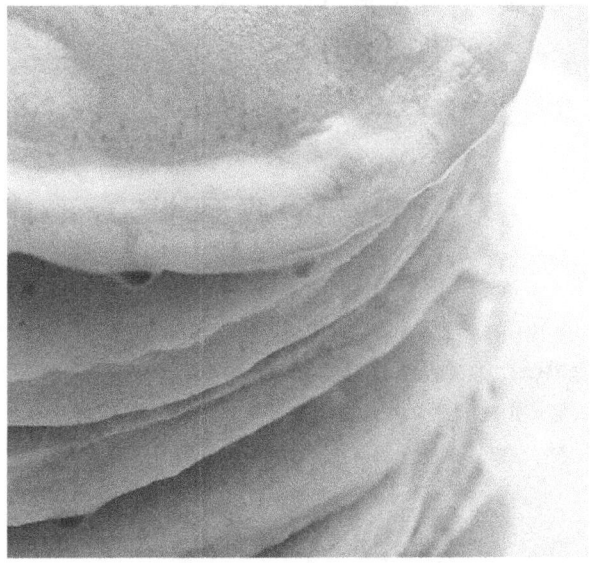

Servings: 4

Ingredients:

- 2 eggs
- ¼ cup of rolled oats
- A pinch of cinnamon
- ½ cup of low-fat cottage cheese

Directions:

1. Crake the eggs into a small bowl and whisk with a fork. Add the oats and cinnamon into the whisked eggs and mix properly to combine. Coat a small non-stick kitchen pan with cooking spray.
2. Place the pan over medium heat, add in the mixture and cook for about two and a half minutes on one side, flip and cook for an additional thirty seconds. Add the cottage cheese and some sprinkles of cinnamon on top. Serve.

Per serving: Calories: 200/ Carbs: 26.8 g/ Fat: 7.8 g/ Protein: 6.7 g

---

Lunch: *Pork and Pineapple Stir-Fry*

This amazing recipe has garlic and ginger which are added to the savory tenderloin to strike a balance in the taste. It is also a great sauce of nutrients which are needed by the body for various functions!

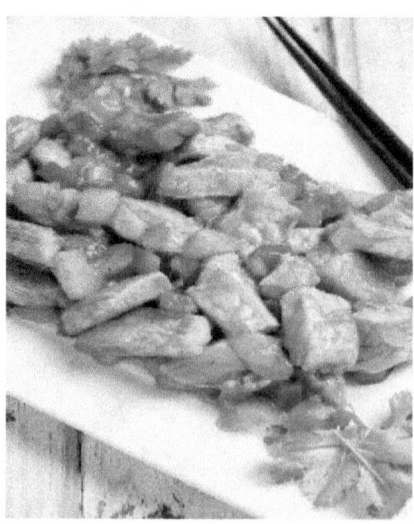

Servings: 4

Ingredients:

- 20 oz. pineapple, cut into chunks
- 24 oz pork tenderloin, cut into chunks
- 1 chopped onion
- 1 tablespoon tapioca starch (optional)
- 1 minced knob of ginger,
- ¼ cup fresh pineapple juice
- 1 chopped big bell pepper
- ¼ cup coconut aminos
- 2 minced garlic cloves
- black pepper, freshly ground
- 2 tbsps. olive oil
- Salt

Directions:

1. Over high heat in a large skillet olive oil.
2. Add pork and stir-fry for 4-5 minutes and place aside.
3. Add onion, ginger and garlic to skillet and cook for 2 minutes.
4. Add pineapple and bell pepper and cook until it's tender.
5. Add in pineapple juice and coconut aminos.
6. Add back the pork and keep on stirring to coat well.
7. Add tapioca starch and stir.

Per serving: Calories: 211/ Carbs: 16.4 g/ Fat: 6.4 g/ Protein: 9.4 g

Dinner: *Creamy Bacon Prawns*

The creamy Bacon prawns recipe is crunchy and delicious recipe. It is filled with nutrition which is good for your health. It has calcium which strengthens your bones and teeth.

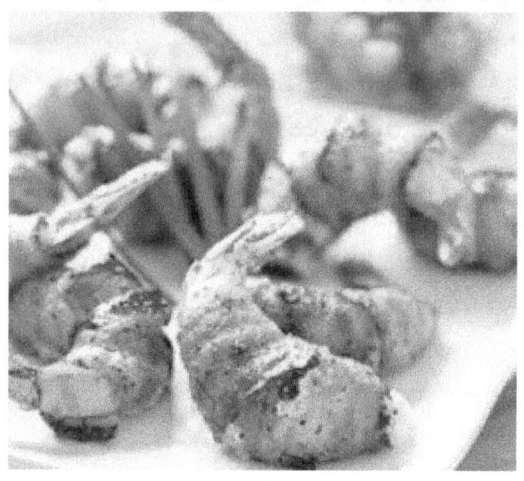

Servings: 4

Ingredients:

- 1lb Prawns
- 1 cup Heavy whipping cream
- Olive oil
- 1 cup Sliced mushrooms
- Freshly ground black pepper
- Chopped chili
- Chopped thyme
- Salt

Directions:

1. Cut bacon into pieces.

2. Set pot to sauté mode then heat and add olive oil and the bacon then cook for 5 minutes or until browned and crispy.
3. Add the sliced mushrooms into the pan then cook for about 5 minutes as you regularly stir.
4. Add prawns and sauté for 2 minutes.
5. Add heavy whipping cream into the pot then add mushrooms and prawns.
6. Add the spices then stir to combine well. Cover the pot and set to cook for 10 minutes over high pressure.
7. Release pressure naturally.
8. Serve and enjoy.

Per serving: Calories 559/ Carbs: 5 g/ Fat: 52 g/ Protein: 21 g

Day 16
Breakfast: *Coconut Flour Pizza*

Cauliflower is an excellent ingredient which aids in weight loss, acts as a good source of antioxidants and rich in sulforaphane. It can be easily added to your diet. The coconut flour contains lauric acid and fiber which makes it very healthy for diabetic patients. It also promotes healthy digestion.

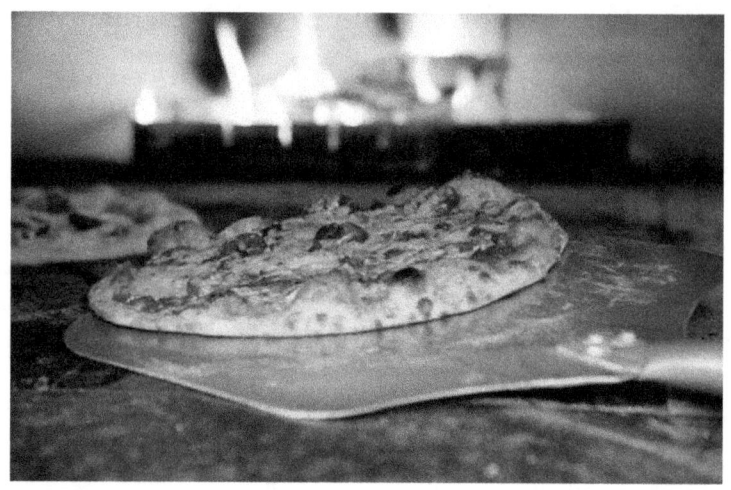

Servings: 2

Ingredients:

- 4 eggs
- 2½ cups cauliflower, grated
- 2 tbsps. coconut flour
- 1 tbsp psyllium husk powder
- ½ tsp salt to taste

Toppings:

- Herbs

- Avocado
- Olive oil
- Spinach
- Smoked salmon

Directions:

1. Preheat the oven to 360 degrees F. Place a parchment paper on a baking sheet pan.
2. Add all the ingredients listed above in a large mixing bowl, one at a time but do not add the toppings. Stir well to combine. Let the mixture sit for about five minutes to thicken up. At the elapse of five minutes, the psyllium and the coconut flour must have absorbed the liquid.
3. Gently pour the pizza base in the lined baking sheet. Make a round shape using clean hands and bake in the preheated oven for about fifteen minutes until the pizza become brown and thoroughly cooked. Once baked, take out of the oven. Serve with desired toppings.

Per Serving: Calories: 454/ Carbs: 26 g/ Fat: 31 g/ Protein: 22 g

---

Lunch: *Instant Pot Turkey Breast*

Turkey is an all-time favorite for many people. It is tasty and will leave you yearning for more. This recipe is better enjoyed with family! Try it today!

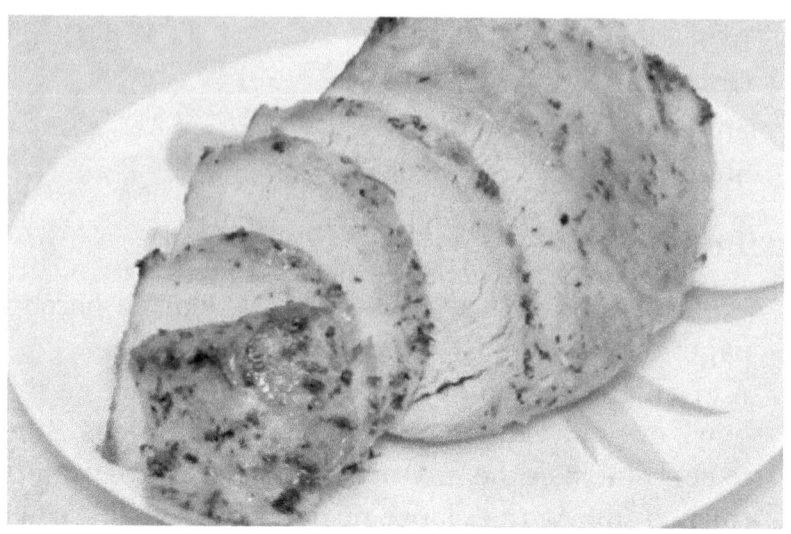

Servings: 2

Ingredients:

- 2 turkey breast fillets
- 1 cup water
- 1 tbsp. Rosemary
- 1 tbsp Garlic powder
- 1 tbsp Sage
- ¼ tsp pepper
- ½ tsp Salt
- ½ tsp Thyme

Directions:

1. Arrange the rack in the Instant Pot or just add the breast to the water for poaching.
2. Use the spices and herbs to rub the turkey and place them into the pot. Secure the lid using the poultry function (7-10 min).

3. Quick release the pressure when the time is done and remove the meat.
4. You can use the juices with the meat or save it for a broth later.

Per Serving: Calories: 268/ Carbs: 9 g/ Fat: 10.7 g/ Protein: 29.9 g

---

Dinner: *Pesto*

This pesto recipe is garlic free and is made with basil and chives for the perfect sauce. It is relatively easier to make compared to many other recipes. Do not forget that is delicious!

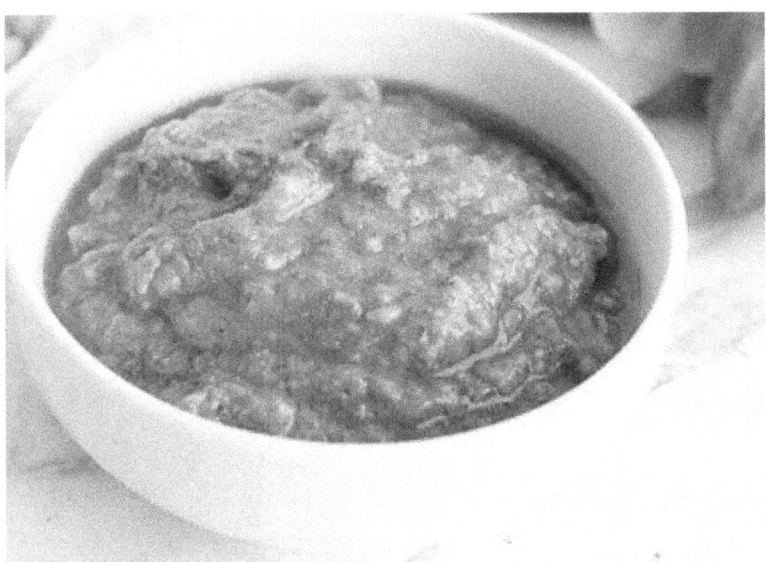

Servings: 2

Ingredients:

- 1 cup chives, chopped
- A squeeze of lemon juice

- ½ cup extra virgin olive oil
- ¼ cup nutritional yeast
- ½ cup grams fresh basil
- ½ cup grams pine nuts
- Salt

Directions:

1. Put all the ingredients in a blender and blend to your wanted pesto consistency. Season with salt and serve.

Per Serving: Calories: 183/ Fat: 19 g/ Carbs: 2 g/ Protein: 2 g/ Fiber: 0.1 g/ Sugar: 2 g

Day 17
Breakfast: *Coconut Flour Waffles*

This meal contains coconut flour which is excellent for diabetic patients as they are low in sugar and high in fiber. They are also low in carbohydrates and contains a lot of proteins which makes them good for weight loss. It contains stevia also which lowers blood pressure and is a sweetener which is good for the teeth.

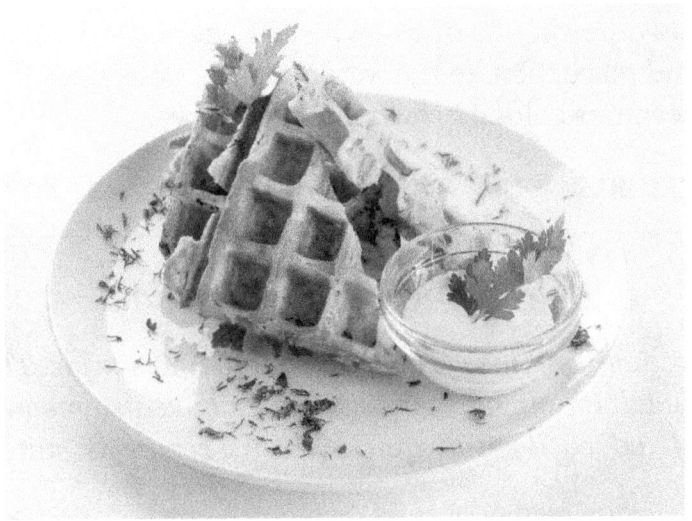

Servings: 4

Ingredients:

- 4 tablespoons coconut flour
- 5 large eggs with the egg whites from the yolks
- 4 tablespoons granulated stevia
- 1 teaspoon baking powder
- 2 teaspoons vanilla extract
- 3 teaspoons full fat milk
- ½ cup melted butter

Directions:

1. In a small mixing bowl, add in the egg yolks, coconut flour, stevia, and baking powder then mix properly to combine. Next, add in the melted butter and mix properly to combine, make sure you attain a smooth consistency. When this is done, add in other ingredients like the milk and vanilla and mix the flour again.

2. Into another mixing bowl, add in the egg whites and whisk with a whisker until it becomes fluffy. Slowly add in some spoons of the whisked egg white into the flour and place them in the waffle maker. Cook until the waffle becomes golden brown in color. Serve.

Per serving: Calories: 278/ Carbs: 7 g/ Fat: 26 g/ Protein: 8 g

---

Lunch: *Coconut Lime Shrimp*

The ingredients of this recipe nourishing and simple. They also taste so well. It only has 5 ingredients which also means that it can be fixed easily and quickly. This recipe is suitable for everyone.

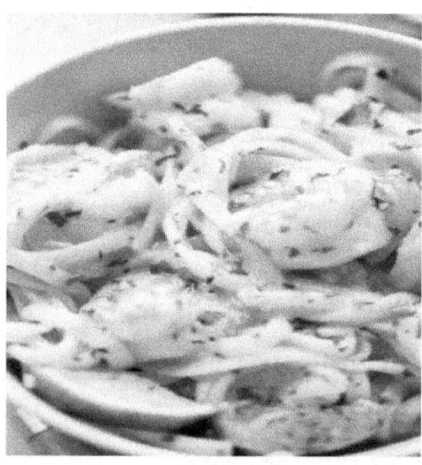

Servings: 3

Ingredients:

- 1/3 cup coconut oil
- 2 pounds large uncooked shrimp
- 1/8 cup honey
- 10 skewer sticks
- 1/3 cup lime juice
- 1 teaspoon salt

Directions:

1. Preheat griddle to medium heat.
2. For every skewer stick, skewer five shrimp.
3. Put the shrimp that you have skewered in a baking dish.
4. Mix salt, honey, lime juice and coconut oil and pour the mixture on the shrimp to coat all skewers.
5. All 15 minutes for the shrimp to marinate.
6. Grill shrimp on each side for 5-6 minutes on the griddle, or until shrimp is firm and white in color.
7. Serve and enjoy.

Per serving: Calories: 421/ Carbs: 42 g/ Fat: 5 g/ Protein: 9 g

Dinner: *Cod with Lemon Caper Spinach*

This recipe is simple and very impressive. It also takes a short time to prepare this recipe. With 20 minutes, the Prosciutto-Wrapped Cod is ready to eat. It also has amazing flavors!

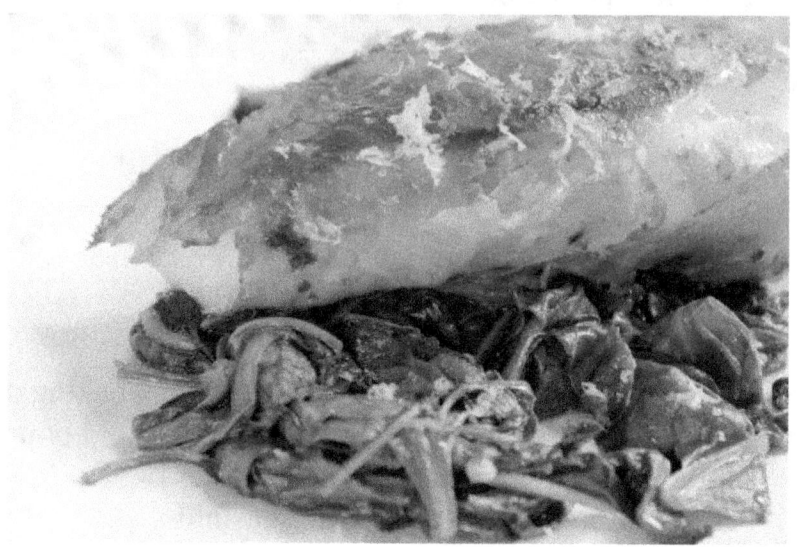

Servings: 2

Ingredients:

- 1.5 ounces prosciutto de parma
- 12 ounces cod fillets
- 3 cups baby spinach
- 2 tablespoons capers
- 1 clove garlic, minced
- Salt
- 2 tablespoons avocado oil
- 1 teaspoon fresh lemon juice
- Pepper
- Zest of 1 lemon

Directions:

1. Use paper towels to pat dry the fillets and let stay for about 30 minutes to come to room temperature.
2. Rub them with pepper and salt.
3. Use prosciutto to wrap the fillets.
4. Heat avocado oil over medium heat in a skillet and add fillets. Cook on each side for 5 minutes, or until fillets are cooked well.
5. Transfer fillets to rack to cool.
6. Stir in the garlic in the pan still on medium heat for 30 seconds. Add lemon juice, capers, and spinach. Stir-cook for 2-3 minutes.
7. Transfer spinach to plates and top with fish. Add some lemon zest and serve.

Per serving: Calories: 354/ Carbs: 23 g/ Fat: 10 g/ Protein: 13 g

Day 18
Breakfast: *Lemon Bars*

This meal contains lemon which is well known for its healthy nutritional values. Lemon is a very good source of vitamin C which protects the immune system from deficiencies and it also acts as a detoxifying agent. The above dish also contains erythritol which is applauded for its nutritional compositions. It is better than sugar and as such it doesn't impair the dental health and it won't lead to diabetes.

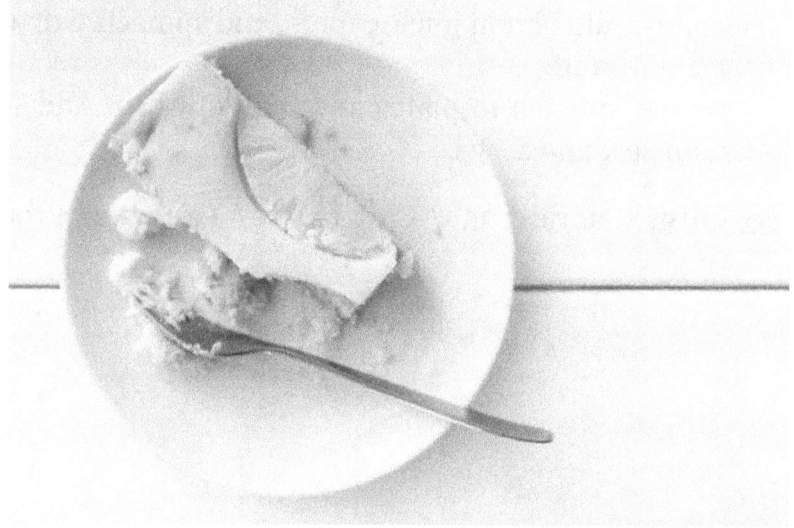

Servings: 3

Ingredients:

- ½ cup of melted butter
- 1¾ cups of almond flour
- 1 cup of powdered erythritol
- 3 medium lemons
- 3 large eggs

Directions:

1. Preheat the oven to three 350 degrees F.
2. In a medium mixing bowl, add in ingredients like one cup of almond flour, a quarter cup of erythritol, and a pinch of salt to taste then stir properly to combine. Place parchment paper on a baking dish then presses the mixture into the dish. Bake in the preheated oven for about twenty to thirty minutes. Once baked, let cool for about ten minutes.
3. In other to make the filling, zest one of the lemons and juice the rest then add into a mixing bowl together with the eggs, erythritol, almond flour and a salt for taste then combine properly. Pour the prepared filling over the crust and bake in the preheated oven for about twenty-five minutes.
4. Serve alongside lemon slices and some sprinkles of erythritol.

Per serving: Calories: 272/ Fat: 26 g/ Carbs: 4 g/ Net Protein: 8 g

---

Lunch: *Balsamic Glazed Salmon*

This Balsamic Glazed Salmon recipe is perfectly cooked to bring out the sweet flavors and healthy nutrients in its ingredients. It can be served alongside favorite side dish. Its ingredients are healthy.

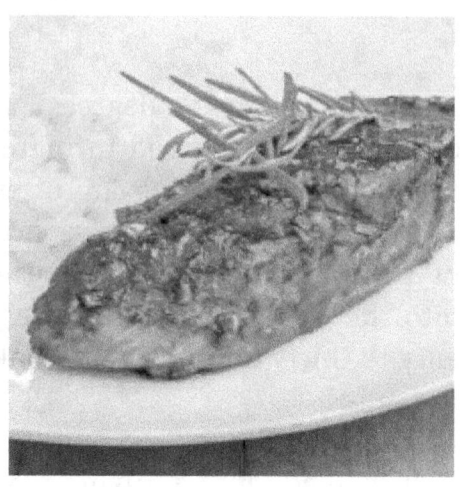

Servings: 4

Ingredients:

- 1/3 cup Balsamic vinegar
- 1-pound salmon
- 2 teaspoons honey
- 1 tablespoon avocado oil
- ½ teaspoon salt
- 2 small cloves garlic, minced
- 1 teaspoon avocado oil

Directions:

1. Preheat oven to 375°F (204°C).
2. Pour avocado oil onto the baking tray and on it put salmon skin side facing down.
3. In a small saucepan, heat avocado oil on medium heat. Add garlic and sauté for about 1 minute. Add pepper, salt, honey and balsamic vinegar and raise heat to high until bubbles are formed. Lower heat to medium and continuously stir for about 3 minutes, or until it starts flaking.

4. Serve and use garnish of your choice.

Per serving: Calories: 402/ Carbs: 28 g/ Fat: 8 g/ Protein: 21 g

---

Dinner: *Plantain Tortillas*

This recipe has very few ingredients and therefore it is very easy to prepare. It is a good nourisher for the body.

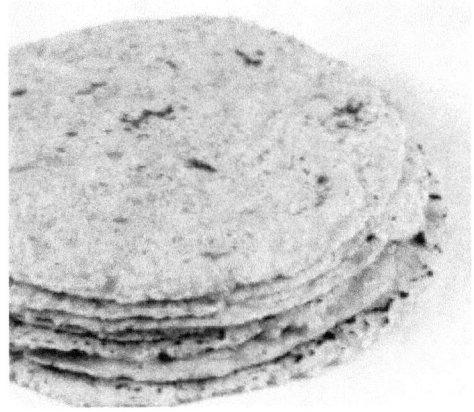

Servings: 4

Ingredients:

- 1 pound peeled, cubed large green plantains
- 1/3 cup water
- 1/3 cup avocado oil

Directions:

1. Preheat oven to 400°F (204°C). Line a parchment paper on two baking sheets and set the rack at the center of oven.
2. Put all ingredients in a blender and blend for 1-2 minutes, starting on low and increasing to high. You may add water to have a thick puree.

3. Divide the batter formed into 12 tortillas and smoothen then on the baking sheets.
4. Bake for about 9-12 minutes and turn the racks. Bake further for about 10-15 minutes more, until they start being brown.
5. Allow to cool for 5 minutes and the serve.

Per serving: Calories: 432/ Carbs: 43 g/ Fat: 10 g/ Protein: 54 g

Day 19
Breakfast: *Cinnamon and Coconut Yogurt*

Due to its healthy fats, coconut butter fills up the body, while the protein from Greek yogurt gives you energy for the day. Cinnamon, on the other hand, has been associated with increased alertness and reduced stress, so one can eat this dish for breakfast right before a big meeting to achieve greater results.

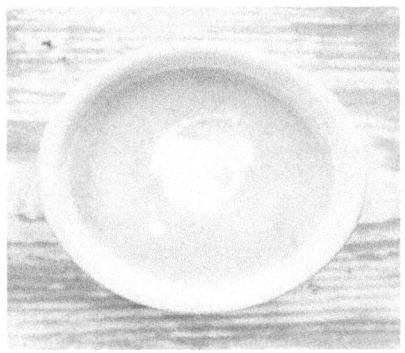

Servings: 1

Ingredients:

- 6 ounces of Greek yogurt
- 1 teaspoon of coconut butter
- 1 tablespoon of shredded unsweetened coconut
- A dash of cinnamon

Directions:

1. Add in the coconut butter and shredded pieces into Greek yogurt then stir properly to combine.
2. Add the cinnamon on top and serve.

Per serving: Calories: 106/ Carbs: 14.8 g/ Fat: 0.1 g/ Protein: 14.1 g

Lunch: *Korean Seafood Pancake (Haemul Pajeon)*

The Korean Seafood Pancakes are delicious recipes made with mixed seafood, cassava flour. If you are looking a perfect seafood, then this is the right one. It is gluten-free and full of energy for you.

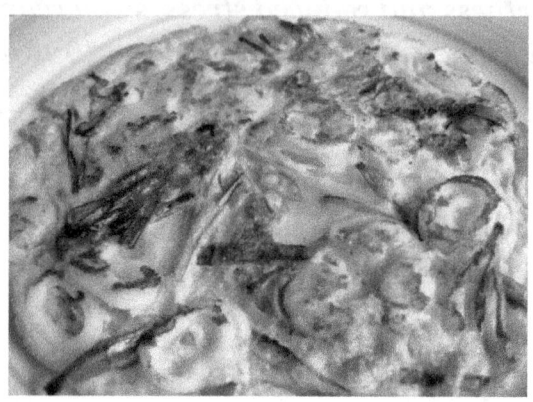

Servings: 4

Ingredients:

- 1½ cups cassava flour
- 2 cups of fresh mixed seafood
- 1 teaspoon salt
- 4 cloves garlic, sliced
- 1¾ cups water
- 2 teaspoon olive oil
- ½ sliced onion
- 1 tablespoon apple cider vinegar
- 1 teaspoon baking soda
- Avocado oil

Directions:

1. Heat a nonstick pan medium heat.

2. Mix seafood mixture, cassava flour, sea salt, baking soda, water, olive oil, onions, garlic and apple cider vinegar to form batter.
3. Use 2 teaspoons avocado oil to grease the pan.
4. Use a cup spoon batter (1 cup) and pour onto the pan and evenly spread it.
5. Cook for 4-5 minutes, or until brown, turn to the other side and repeat. Add more oil as you may need.
6. Once you have finished, cut pancakes into wedges. Serve with coconut aminos and scallions.

Per serving: Calories: 519/ Carbs: 41 g/ Fat: 10g/ Protein: 25 g

---

<u>Dinner:</u> *Beef Bacon Plantain Hash*

You will absolutely love this recipe! If topped with an avocado, it becomes so sweet and delicious. You can as well drizzle some lime juice and cilantro and they make it better!

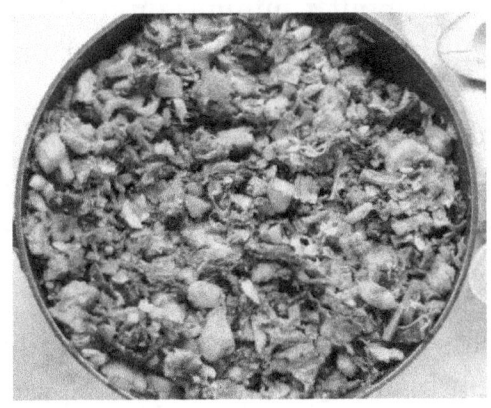

<u>Servings:</u> 5

<u>Ingredients:</u>

- 8 ounces chopped bacon

- juice of 1 lime
- 1 tablespoon garlic, minced
- ¼ cup + ¼ cup chopped cilantro
- 1 pound. grass-fed beef, ground
- 3 peeled yellow plantains, chopped
- 1 teaspoon garlic powder
- 10 ounces brussels sprouts, shredded
- ½ teaspoon salt
- 1 peeled onion, chopped
- 5 ounces chopped kale
- 1½ teaspoons dried oregano
- 2 avocados (optional)

Directions:

1. Over medium heat in a large skillet, cook bacon until crispy. Line a plate with a paper towel and place bacon on it and set aside. Preserve the fat from bacon in a bowl.
2. In a skillet, melt 2 tablespoon bacon fat and sauté plantains for about 5 minutes on medium heat, or until tender and brown. Remove and put on a platter. Set aside.
3. Melt 1 tablespoon of fat from bacon and add garlic and onions and sauté for 2-3 minutes. Add beef and cook until it's brown, or 3 minutes. Add kale and brussels sprouts.
4. Cook for about 3 minutes and cover with a lid until kales and sprouts are tender, about 3 more minutes.
5. Add bacon plantains and also salt, spices, cilantro and lime juice and remove from heat.
6. Top with cilantro and avocado, if you want.

Per serving: Calories: 453/ Carbs: 42 g/ Fat: 16 g/ Protein: 56 g

Day 20
Breakfast: *Keto Greek Yogurt with Peanut Butter*

Greek yogurt is filled with a lot of proteins which reduces body weight and it is also composed of iodine which keeps your weight in check. Due to its high calcium content, it ensures that the body is kept fit. Furthermore, adding Greek yogurt to peanut butter makes it a refreshing breakfast which will keep you healthy and revitalized all through the day.

Unsweetened dark chocolate helps to improve blood flow and lowers blood pressure. It plays a major role too in preventing heart diseases and boost your skin thereby leaving it glowing and healthy.

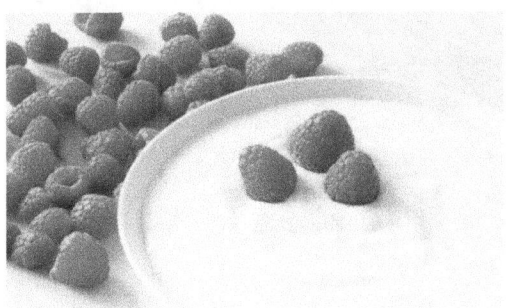

Servings: 1

Ingredients:

- ¾ cup of Greek yogurt
- 1 Pack Dark Chocolate Stick (Unsweetened)
- 1 tbsp. peanut butter
- 1/3 cup strawberries, sliced

Directions:

1. Add the yogurt into a small mixing bowl and then chocolate Stick Pack. Stir to combine.

2. Add the peanut butter onto the mixture. Add the strawberries then serve.

Per serving: Calories: 123/ Carbs: 18.4 g/ Fat: 0.2 g/ Protein: 12 g

---

Lunch: *Pear & Rosemary Stuffed Pork Loin*

Are you looking for a recipe that is festive and fun but still whose maintenance is low? Then this is the recipe you need. It is tasty and it looks beautiful as well! It can be paired with cranberry brussels, wassail or roasted root veggies!

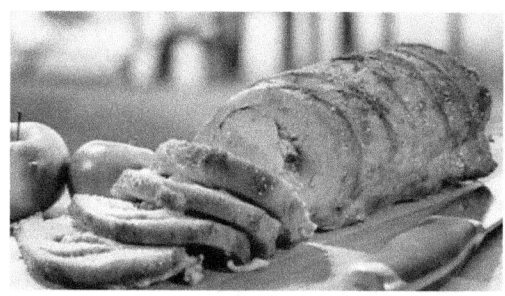

Servings: 3

Ingredients:

- 3 pears, peeled and diced
- 1½ pounds half pork loin, sliced
- Salt
- 1 cup white wine
- 1 large onion, diced
- 3 tablespoons olive Oil (divided)
- 5 fresh rosemary springs

Directions:

1. Preheat oven to 425°F.

2. Heat 2 tablespoons of oil in a medium skillet over medium heat. Add onion and sauté until tender, for 2-3 minutes.
3. Add in pears and the white wine. Allow 10 minutes to simmer without covering.
4. Sin the meantime, spread the pork loin halves and rub with salt.
5. When pears are cooked, stuff the onion and pears into the pork and add rosemary.
6. Use a thread or butcher's twine, tie the pork on 5-6 places and place it on a glass baking dish coated with 1 tablespoon olive oil.
7. Cook for 40minutes to 1 hour while covered with a tin foil. Before serving, let sit for 5 minutes.

Per serving: Calories: 434/ Carbs: 54 g/ Fat: 13 g/ Protein: 43 g

---

<u>Dinner:</u> *Crab Bisque*

Crab Bisque recipe is delicious, comforting, creamy and it is good for your health. It is easy to prepare. The filling soup tastes so nice that you cannot fail to love it.

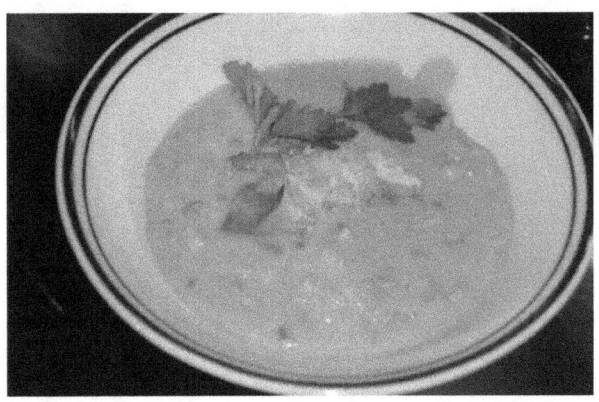

Servings: 6

Ingredients:

- 2 tablespoons avocado oil
- 1-pound cooked crab meat
- 1 (13.5 ounce) can coconut milk
- 1 large coarsely chopped onion
- 1 tablespoon lemon juice
- 4 cups bone broth
- 1½ teaspoons salt
- 2 coarsely chopped cloves garlic
- 1-pound chopped baby carrots
- 2 tablespoons chives

Directions:

1. Over medium heat avocado oil in a large skillet and sauté garlic, onions and carrots for 10 minutes.
2. Add coconut milk and broth and let boil and then lower the heat to low. Allow 10 minutes to simmer while covered, until carrots become tender.
3. Blend the mixture using immersion blender until it is creamy. Add the ingredients that are remaining and heat on stove for a few minutes. Preheat oven to 375°F and coat a 9-inch pie dish with ghee. Set aside.

Per serving: Calories: 521/ Carbs: 36 g/ Fat: 2 g/ Protein: 26 g

Day 21
Breakfast: *Strawberry Shortcakes*

Spice up your day with this sumptuous meal which is very ideal as it helps reduce fats and cholesterol levels leaving you in good shape and fit always. It also consists of fiber and minerals. Maple syrup, on the other hand, is a good substitute for sugar as it improves digestion. It helps prevent cancer and it is good for diabetics so if you love syrup, there is no need to fear as there will be no risk of it increasing your sugar levels.

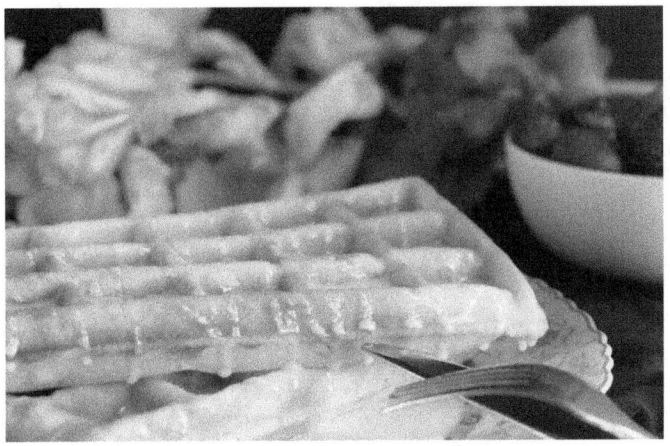

Servings: 2

Ingredients:

- 4 frozen low-fat multigrain waffles
- 1 cup of sliced and fresh strawberries
- ½ cup of plain Greek yogurt
- An adequate amount of Maple syrup

Directions:

1. Make the waffles with directives from the package then place on two serving plates. Add strawberries and yogurt on top then serve alongside maple syrup.

Per serving: Calories: 230/ Carbs: 16 g/ Fat: 1.2 g/ Protein: 7 g

---

Lunch: *Caramelized Salmon*

This is one of the easiest recipes to make. It has only 5 ingredients and only takes only 5 minutes to be ready! It is golden brown and tastes so good and good treat for you and your guests.

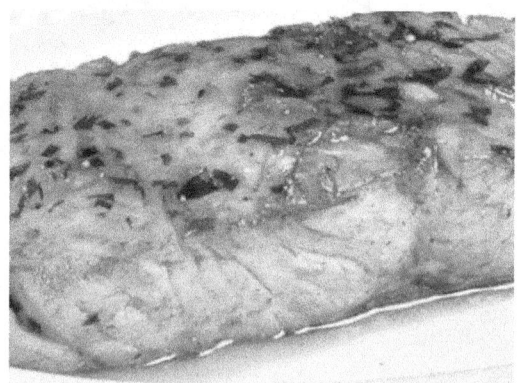

Servings: 1

Ingredients:

- 2 Salmon Filets
- 1 tablespoon sea salt
- ¼ cup coconut sugar
- 2 tablespoons Olive oil
- ¼ teaspoon black pepper (optional)

Directions:

1. Combine pepper, sea salt and coconut sugar in a small bowl.
2. Heat olive oil in a skillet on medium heat.
3. Rub the spice mixture on the salmon fillets.
4. Put the fillets in the pan and cook each side for 2 minutes, or until golden brown and cooked.
5. Serve and enjoy!

Per serving: Calories: 456/ Carbs: 23 g/ Fat: 9 g/ Protein: 32 g

---

Dinner: *Baked Cod*

This recipe is simply delicious! It brings in the best flavor of the cod fillets. It takes few minutes to prepare this amazing recipe. Do not wait any longer as you can prepare this recipe as soon as today!

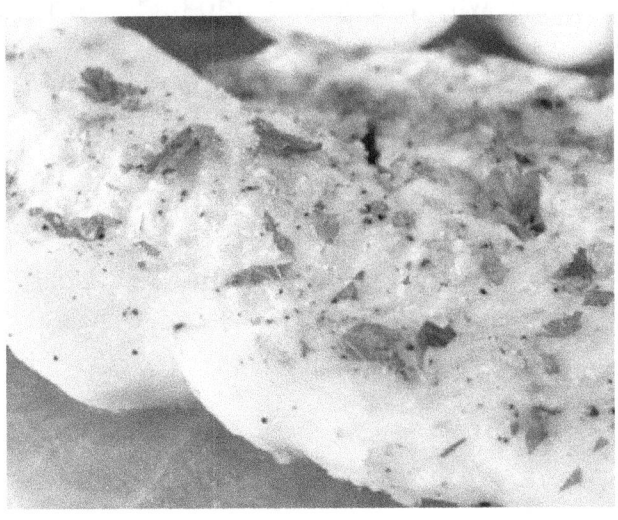

Servings: 3

Ingredients:

- 2oz tomatoes
- Pinch of salt & pepper
- 1 tbsp. chili seasoning mix
- 1 Avocado
- 10oz cod filets, sliced into pieces
- 2 tbsp. melted coconut oil
- 1 tbsp Olive oil

Directions:

1. Add tomatoes in an oven-safe dish. Lay fish pieces over the tomatoes; season with seasoning, salt and pepper and drizzle with melted coconut oil.
2. Add a cup of water in your instant pot and add a trivet.
3. Place the dish in the pot and lock lid; cook on manual for 5 minutes and then let pressure come down on its own. Serve along with peeled avocado on the side and season with olive oil.

Per Serving: Calories: 395/ Carbs: 9 g/ Fat: 14 g/ Protein: 29 g

Day 22
Breakfast: *Frosted Fruit Salad*

The lemon juice in this meal is great as it helps in food digestion. Banana, on the other hand, helps in digestion. Bananas are also referred to as the powerhouse of nutrients and thus making it a great ingredient in this recipe.

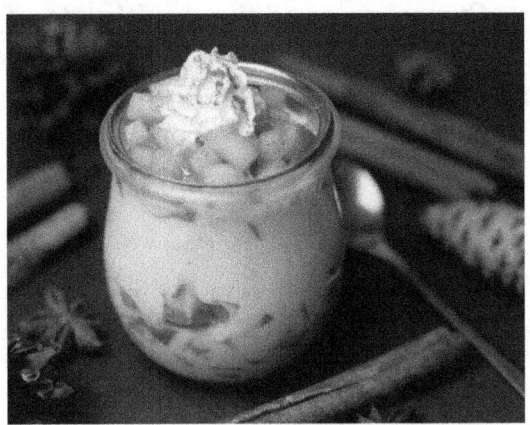

Servings: 1

Ingredients:

- 2 medium sliced firm bananas
- 2 teaspoons of lemon juice
- 1 carton (6 ounces) of fat-free sugar-free raspberry yogurt
- ¼ cup of raisins
- 1 tablespoon of sunflower kernels

Directions:

1. Using a large mixing bowl, add in the apples and bananas, and some sprinkles of lemon juice then toss properly to coat. Add other ingredients like the yogurt,

raisins and sunflower kernels, stir and serve immediately.

Per serving: Calories: 124/ Fat: 1 g/ Carbs: 12 g/ Protein: 3 g

---

Lunch: Thai Whitefish Curry

Thai Whitefish Curry recipe is filled with lots of flavors. It is easy and quick to make as you need only 15 minutes to cook it! You will enjoy its good taste and healthy nutrients.

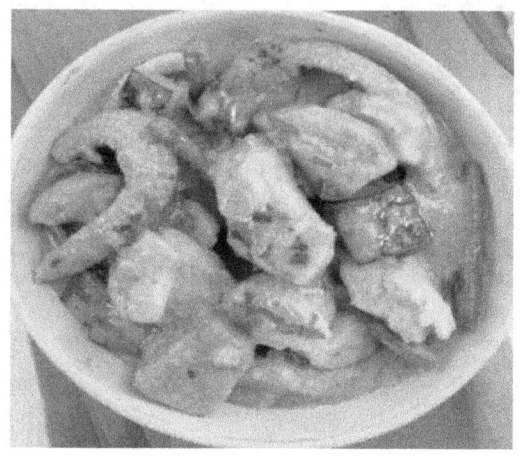

Servings: 4

Ingredients:

- 1-pound white fish
- 2 tablespoons chopped cilantro
- 1cup chopped green onions
- 1 tablespoon ground turmeric
- 2 minced cloves garlic
- 4 teaspoons coconut aminos
- 1 cup sliced shiitake mushrooms
- 1 ½ cups coconut milk

- ¼ teaspoon sea salt
- ½ tablespoon ground cinnamon
- 2 teaspoons ground ginger
- 1 teaspoon coconut oil
- 2 tablespoons lime juice

Directions:

1. Heat coconut oil on medium heat in a skillet. Sear both sides of the fish.
2. Add garlic, ginger, turmeric and cinnamon and cook for one minute.
3. Add green onion and mushrooms and cook fish flakes easily when you use a fork to scratch it.
4. Add in the ingredients that are remaining and heat until ready.

Per serving: Calories: 410/ Carbs: 21 g/ Fat: 24 g/ Protein: 26 g

---

Dinner: *No Bun Hamburger Recipe*

Are you a fan of hamburger? If yes then this is the ideal healthy recipe for you. The only case you would not like this is only if you a vegetarian. This recipe is fixed as it only takes just 10 minutes to cook it making it ideal for a quick lunch for you wherever you could be!

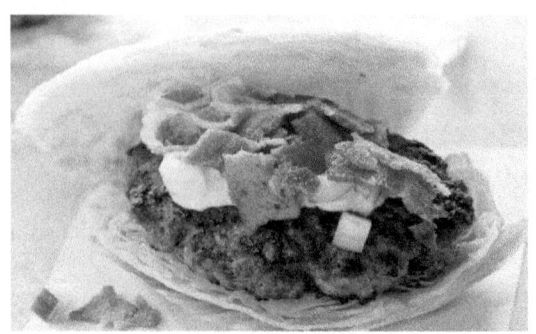

<u>Servings:</u> 6

<u>Ingredients:</u>

For Burgers:

- 2 teaspoons onion powder
- 2 teaspoons garlic powder
- 1 cup mushrooms, minced
- 2 teaspoons paprika
- salt and pepper
- 16 oz ground beef
- 6 slices cheese (if desired)

Toppings:

Top with your favorite burger toppings.

<u>Directions:</u>

1. Mix the patty ingredients in a big bowl. Create individual patties and cook every side for 5-8 minutes in a skillet.
2. Toss lemon juice with arugula and allow 2 minutes to sit before you serve.
3. If you wish, add additional toppings.

<u>Per serving:</u> Calories: 324/ Carbs: 33 g/ Fat: 18 g/ Protein: 53 g

Day 23
Breakfast: *Keto Stuffed Eggs*

This meal contains tabasco which contains 0% fats making it perfect for those abstaining from fats. It also contains mayonnaise which is practically made up of unsaturated fats which helps lower the dangers of high blood cholesterol levels. Mayonnaise also contains vital minerals and vitamins, great for a healthy growth and metabolism.

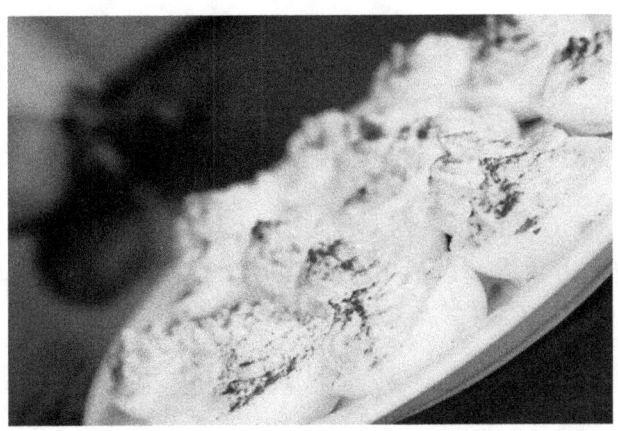

Servings: 4

Ingredients:

- 4 eggs
- 1 teaspoon Tabasco
- ¼ cup mayonnaise
- 1 pinch herbal salt
- 8 cooked, peeled and mashed shrimp or strips of smoked salmon as preferred

Directions:

1. Place a cooking pot over medium heat, add in water and bring to boil.

2. Once the water has boiled, place the eggs gently into the cooking and boil eggs for about eight to ten minutes. Once the eggs are cooked, separate the egg white from its yolk then place the yolks in a small bowl. Mash the yolk with a kitchen folk then add in ingredients like tabasco, herbal salt, and homemade mayonnaise. Combine properly.
3. Add the yolk mixture into the egg whites and place shrimps or salmon on top. Serve.

Per serving: Calories: 163/ Carbs: 0.5 g/ Fat: 15 g/Protein: 7 g

---

Lunch: *Mexican Crab Cakes*

The Mexican Crab Cakes are flour free. They are prepared easily and quickly. It is an amazing recipe and the greatest thing about it is that it is egg free.

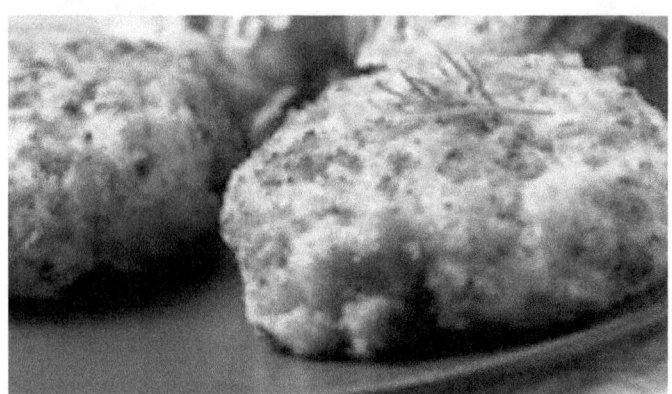

Servings: 4

Ingredients:

- 8 ounces canned crab claw meat
- 3 tablespoons chopped green onion
- ¼ chopped cup cilantro

- 1 teaspoon salt
- 1 tablespoons duck fat
- 1 lime, juiced
- 1 green plantain

Directions:

1. Puree the plantain in a food processor until smooth.
2. Drain crab claw meat and put in mixing bowl.
3. Season with salt and herbs by mixing thoroughly.
4. Mix lime juice and plantain puree together in a small bowl.
5. Use a spatula to fold the mixture into the crab.
6. Divide the mixture into 4 quarter inch cakes.
7. Heat duck fat in a pan over medium heat. Add cakes and cook for 3-4 minutes on each side.
8. Serve on a plate with sauce of your choice.

Per serving: Calories: 432/ Carbs: 31 g/ Fat: 14 g/ Protein: 26 g

---

Dinner: *Chicken Salad Stuffed Peppers*

This meal contains chicken. Chicken is one of the widely consumed meals. It is most especially adored for its sweet taste and low fats and for the fact that it is a lean meat brimming with proteins. It helps to balance the body weight. It aids in the strengthening of the bones in the body and teeth. It is also widely known to be a combatant against all varieties of cancer. The recipe also contains Greek yogurt which is highly rich in proteins. It contains calcium which is ideal for keeping fit and burning fats. Greek yogurt also contains calcium which is cardinal to building strong muscles and aids in the proper functioning of the vital organs.

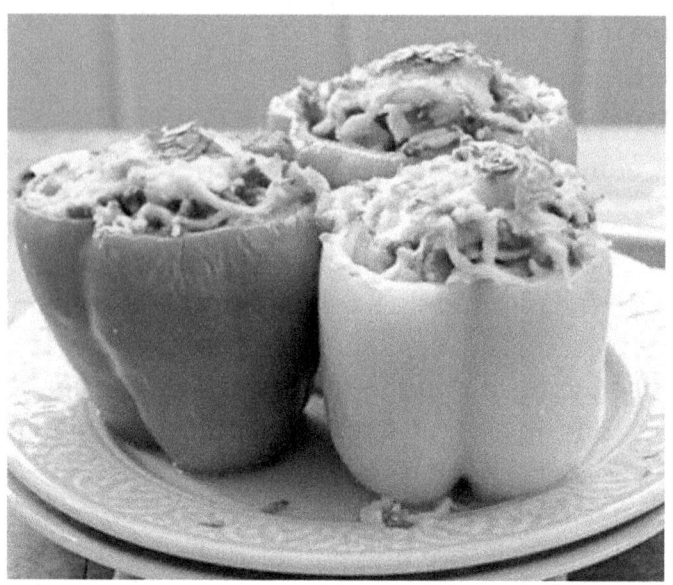

Servings: 3

Ingredients:

- 1 cubed chicken
- 2 tbsps. seasoned rice vinegar
- Salt and ground black pepper
- 2 tbsps. Dijon mustard
- ½ Cup Greek yogurt
- ½ cup fresh parsley, chopped
- 4 stalks of sliced celery
- 1 bunch of sliced and divided scallions
- 1 pint of quartered and divided cherry tomatoes
- ½ diced English cucumber
- 3 halved and seeds removed bell peppers

Directions:

1. Place ingredients like the Greek yogurt, mustard and rice vinegar, salt, and pepper to taste in a medium-sized bowl

and combine properly. Add in the chopped fresh parsley and mix again.

2. Next, to the bowl, ad in ingredients like the chicken, celery, and three-quarters each of the scallions, tomatoes. Add cucumbers then stir everything to combine.
3. Divide the chicken mixture equally among the bell peppers.
4. Place the rest of the scallions, tomatoes, and cucumbers as a garnish on top.

Per serving: Calories: 116/ Fat: 3 g/ Carbs: 16 g/ Protein: 7 g

Day 24
Breakfast: *Egg-In-A-Hole*

The eggs furnish the body with proteins which serve to manufacture body tissues. The Kosher salt is rife with sodium and potassium ions that assist in maintaining the osmotic conditions of the body.

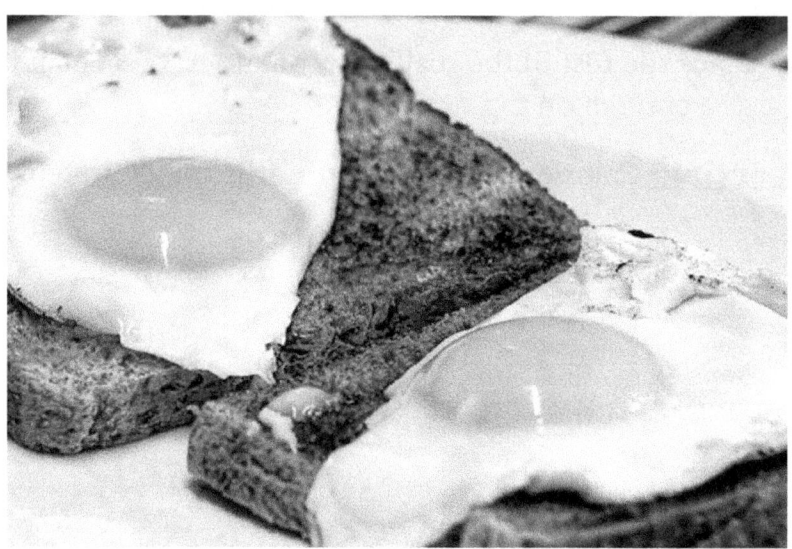

Servings: 3

Ingredients:

- 1/3 cup of mayonnaise
- ¼ cup of grated Parmesan cheese
- 6 slices of toasted bread
- 6 large eggs
- Salt and freshly ground pepper as seasonings for taste
- An adequate amount of hot sauce which is optional

Directions:

1. Place the mayonnaise and cheese in a medium mixing bowl and stir to combine. Spread the mayo mixture equally on each bread toast then use a knife to make holes on each bread toast.
2. Place a large non-stick skillet over medium heat then add in the bread in batches and cook for about one to two minutes on one side then crake an egg into the middle of the bread toast and add salt and pepper for taste. Reduce the heat to low, partially cover the skillet and cook for about one to two minutes until the eggs become set. Serve alongside with the hot sauce and enjoy.

Per serving: Calories: 181/ Carbs: 13.8 g/ Fat: 10.1 g/ Protein: 9.1 g

---

Lunch: *Italian Herb Steak Pinwheels*

This recipe is very simple recipe to make! It is also rich in fresh flavors that make eaters want more of it! The mouthwatering sauce used to coat the flank steak is made up parsley, oregano, pepper and garlic.

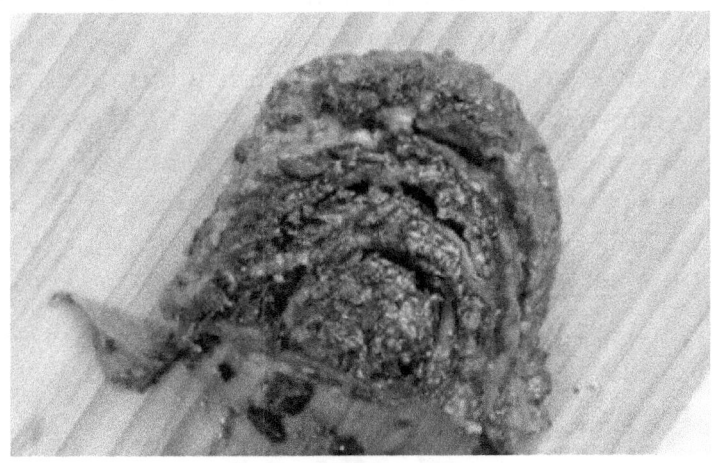

Servings: 8

Ingredients:

- 1-pound flank steak
- 2 tablespoons chopped fresh parsley
- 1 tablespoon extra-virgin olive oil
- red pepper flakes
- avocado oil
- 1 large grated clove garlic
- 1 handful spinach
- 1 tablespoon chopped fresh oregano
- Pepper
- Salt

Directions:

1. Get 8 skewers (wooden) and soak them in water.
2. Preheat oven to medium heat.
3. Cut the steak midway into the thickness almost to edge and unfold to one piece that is flat. Use a mallet to pound the meat under a parchment paper to have a uniform thickness.
4. Rub the meat with garlic and season it with pepper and salt. Top with oregano and parsley and sprinkle olive oil. In a layer over herbs, garlic and meat, arrange spinach.
5. Roll the meat up and use a kitchen twine to secure it. Use pepper and salt to season on the outside. Turn the open side to be up and put in the skewers into the roll.
6. Cut roll into eight 1" thick parts, ensuring that each pinwheel has a skewer.
7. Use avocado oil to oil the grill rack. Grill pinwheels for 3 minutes on each side. Remove from grill and allow about 5 minutes and then serve.

Per serving: Calories: 411/ Carbs: 34 g/ Fat: 11 g/ Protein: 42 g

---

Dinner: *Vegan Fat-Burning Iced Blended Coffee*

What more can one possibly ask for when offered with such an irresistible meal for breakfast. The sweet savor and appealing appearance of this recipe will make you hunger for it as it contains coconut oil, cinnamon and cacao butter which helps to prevent skin dryness and aging. It also improves heart health and improves the immune system of an individual.

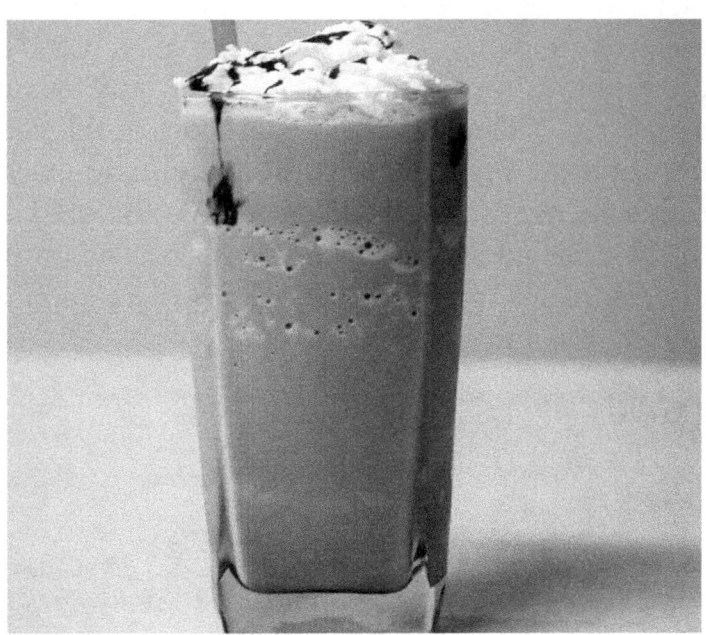

Servings: 1

Ingredients:

- 1½ cup of brewed coffee
- 1 tablespoon of almond butter
- 2 tablespoons of cacao butter

- 1 tablespoon coconut oil as desired
- 4 drops of alcohol-free stevia
- ¼ teaspoon of ground vanilla bean which is optional
- ¼ teaspoon of ground cinnamon which is optional
- 4 ice cubes

Toppings:

- ¼ cup of coconut whipped cream
- 1 teaspoon of cacao nibs

Directions:

1. Place ingredients such as the coffee, almond butter, cacao butter, coconut oil, stevia, vanilla and cinnamon in a high-speed blender or a food processor and blend for a few minutes. Pour the mixture in a jar and place in the fridge to cool off. Once cold, pour the mixture back into the blender, add some cubes of ice and blend until the ice are completely crushed. Add whipped cream and cocoa nibs on top and serve.

Per serving: Calories: 109/ Fat: 3 g/ Carb: 9 g/ Protein: 2 g

Day 25
Breakfast: *Stuffed Avocados*

Mozzarella in the dish contains water-soluble vitamins that supply the immediate nutritional demands of the body. The vitamins are used in the synthesis of red blood cells; maintenance of night vision and a healthy skin. It also provides the body with calcium that hardens the bones. On the other hand, basil prevents the excessive build-up of fats in the liver and maintains its vigor

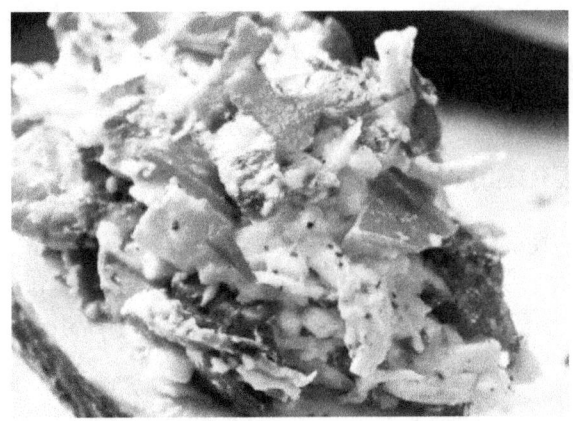

Servings: 2

Ingredients:

- 2 pitted avocados
- ½ cup of halved cherry tomatoes
- ½cup of chopped fresh mozzarella
- An adequate amount of Italian seasoning
- An adequate amount balsamic vinegar
- An adequate amount extra-virgin olive oil
- salt as seasoning to taste
- Freshly ground black pepper as seasoning to taste
- An adequate amount Basil, for garnish

Directions:

1. Scoop out the avocado with the aid of a spoon while leaving a small border. Diced the scooped avocado and place in a medium mixing bowl. In the bowl containing the diced avocado, add in ingredients like the tomatoes, mozzarella, Italian seasoning, balsamic, olive oil, salt, and pepper to taste then combine all to form the salad.
2. Divide the prepared salad among the avocado halves then add basil as garnish. Serve.

Per serving: Calories: 164.2/ Carbs: 11.6 g/ Fat: 11.8 g/ Protein: 15 g

---

Lunch: *Lemon Garlic Pork Chops*

Pork chops rarely disappoint when it comes to delicious taste and nutrition and this recipe is no exception! It can be topped with apples, onions, green veggies or sweet potatoes.

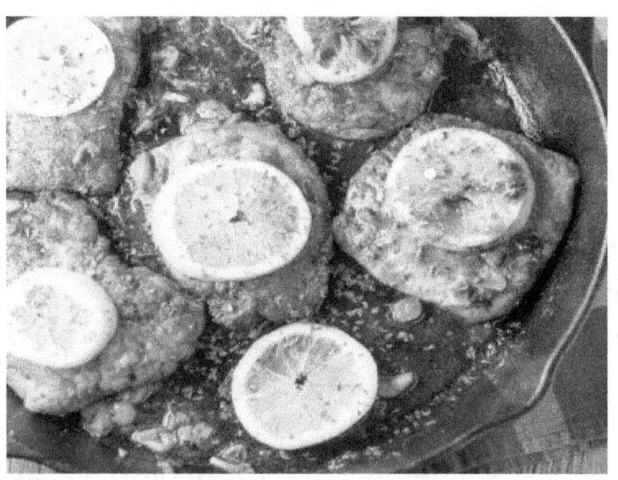

Servings: 3

Ingredients:

- 4 Thin Pork Chops, Skinless & Boneless
- 4 Minced Garlic Cloves
- ¼ Cup Coconut Flour
- 2 Lemons, 1 sliced very thinly and 1 juiced and zested
- 1 tablespoon Olive Oil
- 2 tablespoons Coconut oil
- ¾ cup of bone broth
- 2 tablespoons Fresh Chives, Sliced
- Sea salt
- Black pepper (optional)

Directions:

1. In a shallow bowl, add coconut flour and then stir the lemon zest in. Use pepper and salt to season the pork chops and coat them with coconut flour mixture.
2. Heat oil in a large skillet over medium heat and cook the chops on each side for 3-4 minutes. Remove and put on a plate.
3. Lower heat to medium and add coconut oil and garlic for 30 seconds to 1 minute. Add broth and cook for 4-5 minutes without covering.
4. Return pork chops to pan and the slices of lemon and cook for 2 minutes.
5. Drizzle the lemon juice over and the chives.

Per serving: Calories: 453/ Carbs: 52 g/ Fat: 13 g/ Protein: 36 g

Dinner: *Fat-Burning Keto Latte*

This recipe contains grass-fed collagen which acts as a nutrient that reverses skin aging, helps to build the body muscles and burn fat and improves digestive health.

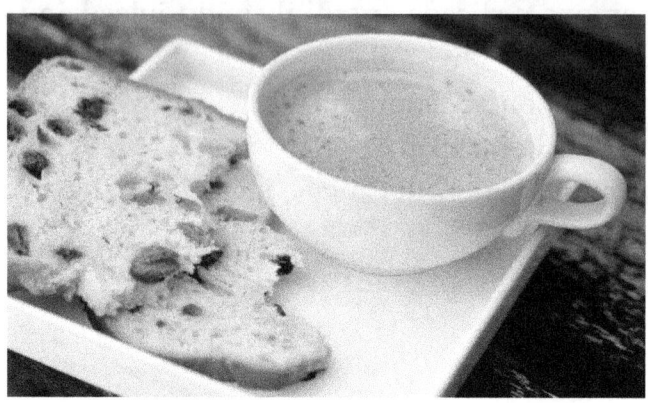

Servings: 1

Ingredients:

- 8 oz. of brewed decaf or regular coffee or tea as desired
- 1 tablespoon of coconut oil is preferred
- 1 tablespoon of cocoa butter
- 1 tablespoon of hemp hearts
- 3 drops of alcohol-free stevia which is optional
- 1 tablespoon of grass-fed collagen

Directions:

1. Make the coffee then place ingredients such as the MCT oil, cacao butter, hemp hearts and stevia in a high-speed blender and blend for about one minute on high. Add the brewed coffee and blend for an addition 10 seconds. Serve.

Per serving: Calories: 136/ Carbs: 11 g/ Fat: 7 g/ Protein: 7 g

Day 26
Breakfast: *Broccoli and Bread Toast*

This beautiful recipe contains a good number of vitamins such as vitamin A and C. It also provides potassium which will make your day filled with savor. Olive oil which we well know is full of proteins and will add a lot of joy to your day when you use it. We are well aware that toasts come in handy as they are healthy, quick and easy to digest.

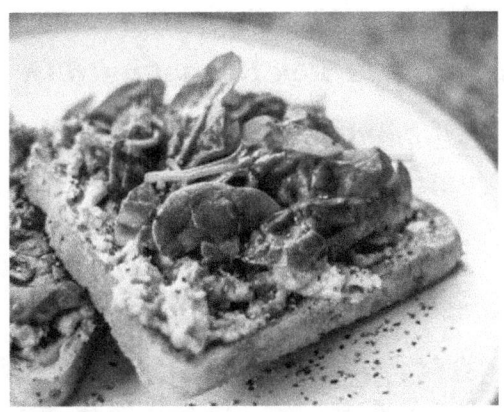

Servings: 1

Ingredients:

- ½cup of broccoli rabe
- 1 teaspoon of olive oil
- 1 slice of red onion
- 1 egg
- 1 slice of sprouted grain bread

Directions:

1. Chop the broccoli with a kitchen knife into small sizes. Place a medium cooking pan over medium heat and add in the oil. Once the oil is hot, add in the onions and

broccoli rabe and cook for a few minutes until the vegetable wilts and becomes aromatic. Remove the cooked broccoli rabe and onion then place the eggs inside the pan and cook until it becomes done. Toast the bread until it attains a golden color then add the vegetable mix and eggs on top. Serve.

Per serving: Calories: 77.2/ Carbs: 4.8 g/ Fat: 5.7 g/ Protein: 3.9 g

---

Lunch: *Pan-Seared Duck Breast with Orange Sauce*

This recipe is definitely so delicious just like many poultry recipes. It is so nutritious with protein, B vitamins, iron, zinc and iron from the duck breast. The oranges are a good source of vitamin C. This recipe can be taken alongside light salad or steamed vegetables

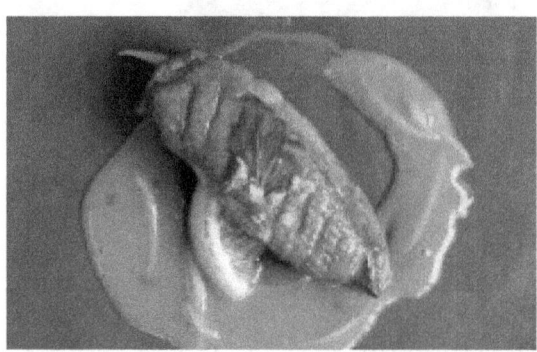

Servings: 2

Ingredients:

- 2 duck breasts, boneless
- ½ cup of chicken broth
- Zest of 1 navel orange
- 2 teaspoons of olive oil, divided

- ½ diced medium onion
- 1 navel orange, Juice squeezed
- ½ Tablespoon of arrowroot flour
- 2 slices of fresh navel orange
- 1 Tablespoon salt
- 2 Tablespoons finely chopped fresh parsley
- Grated orange zest (optional)

Directions:

1. Preheat oven to 285°F (140°C).
2. Score skin and rub salt on the breast to season. In a pan, heat 1 tablespoon olive oil for 1-2 minutes. Sear breasts on high heat with the side with skin facing down until skin is crispy and caramelized. Grease a roasting tray and move the breast on it. With the skin-side up, put it in the oven to cook as you finish up the rest.
3. Grill 2 slices of orange in the pan for garnishing. Set aside.
4. For sauce, add the remaining olive oil to the pan and sauté onions until golden brown. Deglaze by adding orange juice and also the orange zest. Cook for 1-2 minutes and remove from heat. Sieve the sauce through a mesh sieve and throw away the onions and leaving the muslin.
5. Heat the sieved sauce and add the zest strips. In a jug, whisk in arrowroot to the stock and pour the mixture into a pan and cook until it is sufficiently thick.
6. Serve and garnish with grated orange zest, grilled orange garnish and parsley.

Per serving: Calories: 442/ Carbs: 43 g/ Fat: 16 g/ Protein: 54 g

Dinner: *Adobo Chicken Burgers*

The Adobo Chicken Burgers recipe is so much full of flavor and very juicy. The turmeric brings in a sweet flavor and makes it crunchy and healthy. It is easily and quickly prepared as it takes only 10 minutes.

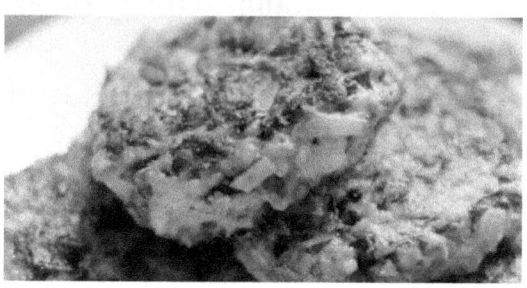

Servings: 6

Ingredients:

- 1-pound ground chicken
- 1 tablespoon Seasoning
- 1 cup finely chopped spinach
- 2 teaspoon ghee
- ¼ cup finely diced onion
- 1 teaspoon salt

Directions:

1. Preheat oil in a large skillet over medium heat.
2. Mix spinach, onion, seasoning and chicken in a bowl to combine. Split the mixture into 6 equal bugger patties.
3. Cook the patties each side for about 4-5 minutes.
4. Serve over lettuce wrap, bed of spinach or roasted veggies.

Per serving: Calories: 530/ Carbs: 25 g/ Fat: 12 g/ Protein: 53 g

Day 27
Breakfast: *Bacon and Lettuce Breakfast*

This meal contains a lot of lettuce which is good for weight loss as it includes a lot of water contents loaded with minerals and vitamins. It also helps control the PH level of the body. The meal also contains avocado pear which includes healthy monosaturated fatty acids and vitamins that aids in weight loss.

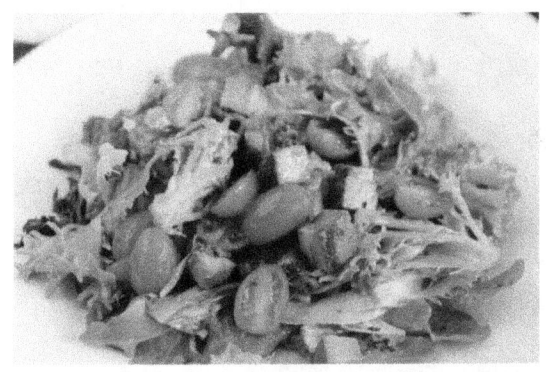

Servings: 1

Ingredients:

- 1 tablespoon of Brain Octane Oil
- ¼ teaspoon salt
- ¼ cup chopped organic romaine lettuce
- 2 slices cooked bacon
- 2 slices tomatoes
- 1 avocado, sliced and mashed
- Micro cilantro

Directions:

1. In a small mixing bowl, add in ingredients like the mashed avocado, one tablespoon of Brain Octane Oil,

and Himalayan pink salt then mix them properly to combine.

2. Place the romaine lettuce on a serving plate then top with the mashed avocado mixture. Place the slices of cooked bacon on top. Next, add in the micro cilantro and a small sprinkle of Himalayan pink salt to taste. Garnish with tomato slices and serve.

Per serving: Calories: 387/ Carbs: 9 g/ Fat: 35 g/ Protein: 11 g

---

Lunch: *Beef 'Goulash'*

This hearty and hot recipe is good for dinner stew. This is a staple Hungarian recipe and it has become popular in many parts of the world. With this recipe, you can use your favorite vegetable as it goes well with vegetables!

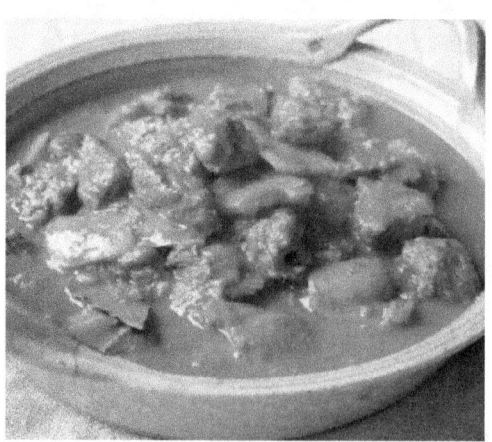

Servings: 1

Ingredients:

- 1-pound diced beef roast
- 4 Tablespoons avocado oil
- 10 quartered white button mushrooms

- 4 peeled cloves garlic, chopped
- 1 teaspoon turmeric
- 1 peeled medium onion, chopped
- 1 cup bone broth
- 2 Tablespoons chopped fresh parsley
- 2 diced carrots
- 1 Tablespoon arrowroot powder (optional)
- Salt

Directions:

1. In a pan, heat olive oil. Add garlic and onion and sauté until tender. Add beef and cook until brown. Add in carrots and mushrooms and cook for about 4-5 minutes.
2. Lower heat to low and add beef stock. Allow 60 minutes to simmer while covered with a pan and occasionally stirring. To avoid catching of the mixture, you may add some water.
3. Cook the meat until it is soft and the sauce is thick.
4. To thicken further, add arrowroot powder. Season with salt.
5. Serve over mashed cauliflower or cauliflower rice and use parsley to garnish.

Per serving: Calories: 342/ Carbs: 21 g/ Fat: 16 g/ Protein: 46 g

---

Dinner: *Low carb cheese burger wraps*

This Do-not-forget recipe is not only delicious but it is also tender and can be made easily. It is also comforting food and the greatest thing about it is that it is dairy free and low carb! Try it today and you will not be disappointed!

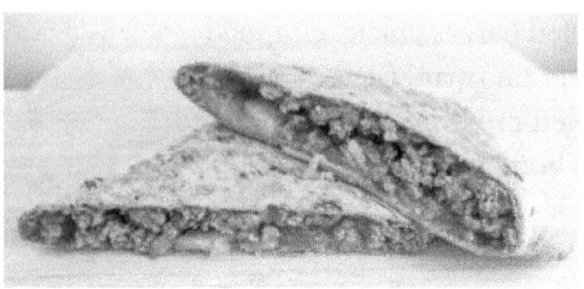

Servings: 4

Ingredients:

- 7 oz Bacon
- 4oz Sliced mushrooms
- 1½ lbs. Ground beef
- 1 cup Shredded cheddar cheese
- ½ teaspoon Salt and pepper
- 1 Iceberg lettuce

Directions:

1. Place a large skillet over medium heat then add bacon and cook to the desired crispiness. Remove from the pan once cooked then set aside.
2. Add mushrooms to the pan then sauté until tender and browned for about 7 minutes then remove from the pan and set aside.
3. Add ground beef then season with salt and pepper. Sauté until cooked well for 10 minutes and use the back of a wooden spoon to break the chunks.
4. Spoon ground beef into the lettuce leaves then sprinkle with cheddar cheese as you also top with bacon and mushrooms.

Per serving: Calories: 584/ Carbs: 5 g/ Fat: 16 g/ Protein: 48 g

Day 28
Breakfast: *Strawberry Smoothie*

This meal contains strawberries which are a great source of fiber, vitamin C and antioxidants which lowers blood pressure, improve immune functions, treats arthritis and cancer, and regulates blood sugar and a lot more. It also contains spinach which is well loaded with vitamins and minerals making it ideal to control the PH level of the body.

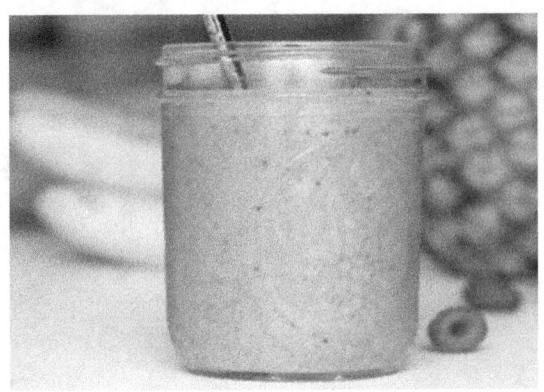

Servings: 2

Ingredients:

- 2 cups of frozen strawberries
- 2 cups of coconut milk
- 1 cup of baby spinach
- ½ freshly squeezed orange juice

Directions

1. Place all the ingredients in a food processor or a blender and blend until it becomes smooth. Serve in cups.

Per serving: Calories: 394.4/ Carbs: 11.6 g/ Fat: 40 g/ Protein: 4.43 g

Lunch: *Plantain Carnitas Nachos*

This recipe does not contain any grains. Instead of chips, this recipe is prepared using green plantains. They are crispy sweet and good for everyone. You will enjoy them

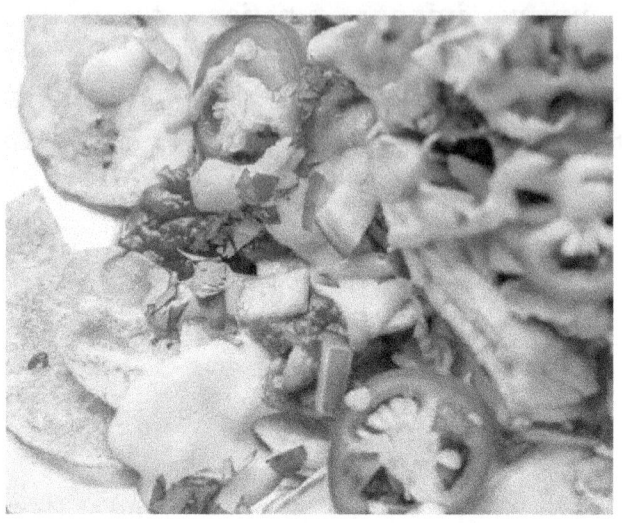

Servings: 2

Ingredients:

- 2 sliced large green plantains
- 2 tablespoons coconut oil
- Avocado lime sauce, 2 servings
- 3 tablespoons fresh cilantro
- ¼ cup red onion
- 1 teaspoon sea salt
- Pork carnitas, 2 servings
- Juice of ½ lime

Directions:

1. On medium heat, melt coconut oil in a skillet. And add the plantain.
2. Sauté until lightly brown and tender.
3. Remove from heat.
4. Use a glass cup bottom to smash and flatten the plantain.
5. Return the plantains to the oil.
6. Get the green plantains and place in a big plate.
7. Start to layer avocado lime sauce, cilantro on the carnitas.
8. Use extra lime to top, if needed.

Per serving: Calories: 299/ Carbs: 14 g/ Fat: 13 g/ Protein: 32 g

---

Dinner: *Avocado Egg Salad*

Avocados are loaded with a lot of healthy monosaturated fatty acids good for lowering cholesterol and triglyceride levels resulting in healthy growth. As for lime juice, it is well known that it is very good for digestion as it helps the saliva break down food for better digestion. It also contains acidity which is good for clearing the excretory system.

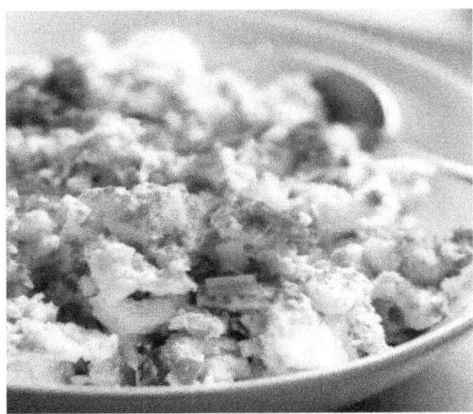

Servings: 4

Ingredients:

- 4 large and diced hard-boiled eggs
- 1 diced avocado
- 2 green and sliced onions
- 4 slices of cooked and crumbled low-sodium bacon
- ¼ cup of plain yogurt
- 1 tablespoon of low-fat sour cream
- 1 whole lime juice
- 1 tablespoon of snipped fresh dill
- ¼ teaspoon of salt
- 1/8 teaspoon of fresh ground pepper

Directions:

1. Place the eggs in a muffin pan then place in the oven to hard-boil the egg. The oven should be set at 325 degrees F.
2. Once the egg is hard-boiled, place in cold water for a few minutes then peel off the shells. In a large salad bowl, add in the eggs and other ingredients like the avocado, green onions, and bacon then combine properly and set aside.
3. Using a large mixing bowl, add in ingredients like the yogurt, sour cream, lime juice, dill, salt, and pepper to taste and whisk together to combine using a whisker.
4. Add in the yogurt mixture into the bowl containing the egg mixture and stir properly.
5. Add dill and crumbles bacon as a garnish then serve.

Per serving: Calories: 269/ Carbs: 8 g/ Fat: 21 g/ Protein: 11 g

Conclusion

Thank you for taking the time to read the book *Intermittent Fasting*. Many people struggle with dieting plans and getting one that's capable of providing the desired results have always been a challenge. One thing that makes Intermittent fasting to be significant is the fact that fasting is a practice that comes so naturally to the body. It's easy to start fasting and flexible to sustain as you don't have to worry about the foods that you eat and the macronutrients.

I know that you have found valuable information regarding what Intermittent fasting entails and how you can make use of it for optimal health and weight loss. Intermittent fasting doesn't have to be a struggle if you choose the right fasting protocol that suits you best and goes by the guidelines.

It's important to note that intermittent fasting is not a quick fix. You will not automatically lose weight just because you are fasting. You also have to watch your diet and ensure that the foods that you consume are helping you towards realizing your desired goal.

www.ingramcontent.com/pod-product-compliance
Lightning Source LLC
Chambersburg PA
CBHW060848170526
45158CB00001B/279